The Lottery

John MacCusack

AuthorHouse™ UK Ltd.
500 Avebury Boulevard
Central Milton Keynes, MK9 2BE
www.authorhouse.co.uk
Phone: 08001974150

© 2011 John MacCusack. All rights reserved.

No part of this book may be reproduced, stored in
a retrieval system, or transmitted by any means
without the written permission of the author.

First published by AuthorHouse 3/7/2011

ISBN: 978-1-4567-7407-3 (sc)

Any people depicted in stock imagery provided by Thinkstock are models,
and such images are being used for illustrative purposes only.
Certain stock imagery © Thinkstock.

This book is printed on acid-free paper.

Because of the dynamic nature of the Internet, any web addresses or
links contained in this book may have changed since publication and
may no longer be valid. The views expressed in this work are solely those
of the author and do not necessarily reflect the views of the publisher,
and the publisher hereby disclaims any responsibility for them.

For Anna, Luke, Erin and Zach.

Roger Williams was driving home from work for the last time as he was forced to take early retirement. He was thinking of his life as a child, his love for mathematics and of great expectations during his working life. He remembered taking the same route home about thirteen years ago when his son was only six years old. But on that occasion his enthusiasm was at its peak. He might as well have been on cloud nine then.

At the College where he had been employed as a mathematics teacher for nine years, he was, on that day, appointed as head of Department of Mathematics. He had been short-listed a number of times in the past but, for some reason, he was never the final choice. This time the position required more work than ever and for the first time the headship did not bring any financial rewards and, possibly for these reasons, he was the only candidate.

Roger himself saw it as a recognition of his abilities and was very proud of himself. He was finishing his sandwich during his lunch break, still seeing himself as the Head of the Maths Department for years to come, when his wife, Amanda, phoned to tell him that Mathew, their son, had won the annual mathematics competition for bright young mathematics enthusiasts. The committee members called Mathew for an interview before awarding him the first prize because they had never had a test result with such high marks.

Roger's mind went back to the time when he was a young boy of 12 and had won the same competition and was so proud of himself. But what was so special here was that Mathew had just had his sixth birthday, and the tests in both cases were of the same standard. That was, probably the point in time when Roger's life changed direction.

'Amy, I am taking you out tonight, to celebrate something special' said Roger as he entered the kitchen where his wife was preparing the dinner. He did not tell her the news about the appointment when she phoned at lunchtime because he wanted to enjoy the feeling of joy for himself for as long as possible.

'No Roger, not tonight. I am cooking a special meal for Mathew, for his success in the mathematics competition. Anyhow, what could be more special today than Mathew's achievement. He is such a bright boy. Don't you think so?'

The correct word would be genius but, by now, Roger was so deflated by no response from his wife, although he did not tell her about his promotion at the college, that he went upstairs and stayed in his study until a shout came from downstairs that the dinner was ready.

When Mathew was called for the interview and

subsequently awarded the first prize, he felt no elation and happiness and the only thing he thought was of his father and how his father will react towards him. His father, on the other hand could not get his wife to ask him about the "something special" that he mentioned earlier. The atmosphere, during the dinner, was somewhat quiet and soon Mathew excused himself and went to his bedroom saying he felt a bit tired. He was actually annoyed that his father did not ask him much about the competition and thought that the maths prize was probably not such a big thing.

Amanda, on the other hand, was so proud of what their son Mathew achieved that all their relatives and neighbours new of Mathew's success the very next morning.

Williams's family lived in a small town of Lowestry situated at the England – Wales border. Roger drove each day about fifteen miles to his college and Mathew had about twenty minutes ride on the school bus. Those in Lowestry who new the Williams family said how proud they must be. Some of the neighbours however thought that Mathew would be better off if he mixed, at least a bit, with other boys and got involved with sports, because he looked weak and pale as if lacking even fresh air and was quite small for his age.

But Mathew not only disliked sports. He did not

know why but, he preferred to think about a problem and then try to solve it in his head. That was for Mathew the activity he craved for. Even at the age of six, his bedroom was tidy, bookshelves in order and on his writing desk everything had its own place.

On his fourth birthday his father brought home a computer and as Mathew showed an interest, he was allowed to watch his father work, preparing next day's lectures and test sheets for students. By the age of six, Mathew was able to get out of the computer more than an average adult could. Roger was so proud of his son that he often pretended to be thinking aloud and getting stuck at the particular problem in order to give Mathew a chance to think and come out with an answer.

Mathew never guessed but always thought deeply before giving the correct result. Those were the happiest days in Roger's life since he himself won that mathematics test all those years ago, and for Mathew, he thought that things could only get better.

There were anxious times before he and Amanda brought Mathew home from the hospital, as he was very delicate as a baby, very small and looked as if he was born prematurely.

It took two years before Mathew could walk and even then he preferred to be carried or sitting in his push chair looking at the children's books on his lap.

His mother used to read to him, books containing pictures of animals and their names written underneath.

One day she noticed that he was saying words like "cat" and "dog" while pointing to the text as if he was reading the words themselves.

'Doctor do you think that a child of two could recognize words written in the book?' asked Amanda when she took Mathew to the doctor to get something for his cold and sore throat.

'No Mrs Williams' said Dr Johnston; baby's brain cannot process such complex information. May be in a year or so but for now why don't you give him colouring in books and let him play with colours. This will improve his hand coordination and it will definitely give him more pleasure.'

The very next day Amanda replaced all the books containing words by the colouring in ones but she still read Mathew stories at bedtimes. She wasn't sure whether Mathew was listening but he fell asleep much quicker when a story was read to him.

'Roger come and see this please' shouted Amanda holding a picture book in her hand.

Her husband rushed from the TV room thinking there was something wrong and was almost crossed with her seeing that everything was orderly.

'Look at this Roger, Mathew wrote this' said Amanda half scarred hearing what she had just said.

'Mathew probably copied it from a book Amy. You know how clever children can be.'

But Roger, I put away all the books that have any letters in them and gave Mathew only picture books to colour in as the doctor suggested.'

Roger stood there in the middle of the sitting room and tried to "solve" the puzzle.

'If Mathew did write that down from his head, he should be able to do it again.'

So he asked Amanda what animals their son knows by name and then prepared the test. They sat down and Mathew was given a pencil and a picture book and asked to write under the picture as his mother had thought him.

For a while it looked as if Mathew did not even understand what he was supposed to do and then he started writing. The letters were bad, of course, but eventually he did write: cat, dog, cow, and sheep under the appropriate pictures.

There was silence in the room until Amanda jumped and gave Mathew a huge hug, which Mathew rejected by turning his head back towards the book. He felt uneasy when his mother did that. He did not like any body contact.

Now and then Roger and Amanda had visitors for dinner, mostly Roger's colleagues from the College. There was John Davidson, teaching applied mathematics, very able young man but, when he was outside the college, he was a dedicated sports fanatic. Then there was Tom Montgomery, who was older than Roger and got his Phd in Cambridge where he carried out research in abstract mathematics, a very obscure field, so much so that he never did any work in that field since taking the post at the college.

They enjoyed coming because of Amanda's Italian cooking. After dinner they used to present teasers in mental problem solving. If it was not too late, Mathew was allowed to sit on the corner sofa and listen.

He absorbed every word said. On one of those occasions, Mathew was just seven years old, when one of Roger's colleagues presented them with the question teaser of "five hats"

'Three clever men are standing, one behind the other in a darkened room', started John Davidson. 'A hat, of random selection from three white and two black hats, is placed on each man's head. The two remaining hats are then removed from the room. When the lights are switched on, the last man in the row sees the two hats on the heads in front of him. The second man sees only the one hat in front of him while the man in front sees no hats at tall.

One of the men has to guess what is the colour of the hat he has on his head. After a while the man in front says: "I have a white hat". How did he come to that conclusion'?

Mathew, with paper and pencil on his lap, tried to put all the data down as fast as he could.

The answers varied with solutions such as "not possible" or "pure luck" until Mathew said:

'I know'… it is really very simple' They all turned their heads and Roger regretted letting Mathew stay because if his son comes up with a silly answer he, Roger, will look silly as well because he always talked how Mathew can do this or do that and now all that could collapse.

At least that was how Roger felt. But he was surprised with the delight of his colleagues asking the boy for his answer.

Mathew said: 'The man at the back does not see two black hats and could not give the correct answer about himself. The man in the middle thinks: If the hat in front of me was black I could say that I have a white hat otherwise the man behind me could say he has a white one. But as it is not, I could not answer. The man in front goes through the thoughts of the two men behind him and says: "I have a white hat". It could not be any other way' said Mathew.

There was silence in the room. Roger's guests were amazed with the way Mathew could analyse the problem and wandering as to what kind of mind that young boy had, and Roger for the first time, became jealous of his son.

'He will be replacing you very soon in the college, Roger, that is something we have never seen or heard of before. Your son can reason and think mathematically better than our gifted students'.

Roger was so confused in his mind and he did not know how to behave towards his son any more. He could not treat him as a child any more, not after the explanation about the hats and yet he could not treat him as an adult, not at the age of seven.

'Darling you were brilliant. You were so fast, I could hardly follow you with my eyes on the track and you left all the boys well behind,' said Ann to her son Joe at the end of the school's sports day where he competed in his local primary school's one hundred metres run.

His father, Paul, did not say anything but he was so proud that he felt twice as tall as his 6ft 1in stature; and why not? Joe was only five and the run was a final, after three pre qualifying runs and Joe won all of them. And more than that, all the other boys in the final run were twice his age.

Paul Brown, his wife Ann and their son Joe lived in Manortown, Cheshire, in the house they bought for cash after Paul's parents died and Paul had sold the inherited house wanting to move away just before he and his wife Ann decided to have children.

Joe was built like a bulldog. Even since he started to walk, and his proud father took him for a stroll, Joe would run, holding his father's hand and soon he was able to run on his own, his father just being able to keep pace.

Paul enjoyed going to the park and meet other parents with their children of similar ages. He would sit on the bench and glow with pride witnessing his son's acrobatics and wandering back to the time when he, Paul, was small and wanted to play with other children. He had three sisters and two brothers, himself being the eldest and in order to help the family budget, he had to earn money since he could remember.

Because of that, there was no time for play and for proper sporting activities with other boys. But he had brains and managed to get a good education and became a chartered accountant. The money he earned was more than many of his and his wife's friends earned as couples.

As time passed, Ann and Paul noticed and had to admit to themselves that Joe was really slow in any mental work. At the age of five when Joe started primary school and the children were tested, his IQ was so low, that Ann and Paul decided they better give him a head start in sport especially when he was physically so strong and healthy.

The group sport did not appeal to them as Joe always preferred to be alone, so the first thing Paul did was to take Joe to his golf club and show his son what was there.

'Dad, I would like to play tennis if that is all right with you'

'Of course son, I will book us a time slot here and we can try and see how you like it.' 'We can try a few other sports as well added Ann.'

'But I do like it Dad, I played in school and can hit the ball well.'

Paul tried and was able to get a booking for first thing in the morning when the tennis court would be empty and they went home. The next day the whole family went to the golf club and Paul and Joe started to hit the ball. Joe's racket was small but still big enough for a child of five. After about half an hour Paul told Joe to go and have a shower and he turned to Ann and they, without saying anything, agreed that Joe is a natural and that was that.

'Mrs Taylor, your son is not ill but has some kind of genetic immunodeficiency and we are afraid that he will always be prone to catch any disease he gets in contact with,' said Dr Hearn.

That does not mean that Tom could not lead as normal life, as any other child providing he does not over exert himself.'

'"Genetic immunodeficiency" the doctor said', Tom's mother Irene was explaining to her husband Steve. 'Is it because we are doing something wrong or Tom needs more sun and fresh air?'

'No Irene, children are all different and he will grow out of it when he gets a bit older.

If there was something wrong with him, we would have been told by now.'

'You talk as if there is something wrong with him.'

'On the contrary. I think Tom will be as normal as you and me.'

Irene Taylor took Tom to the specialist because of child's slow progress both mentally and physically. They had to travel by bus and by train to Birmingham because Irene did not drive and the town Cranspole, just south of Cheltenham where Steve and Irene Taylor lived with their son Tom had no resident specialist that was to examine Tom.

Tom was almost two when he started attempting to

walk, was rather small for his age but enjoyed music and would listen and tap with his hands when his mother played a tune on the piano. Sometimes she felt that he recognized the tune almost immediately if he heard it being played previously.

With his dark hair and very light blue eyes on his tiny pale face, Tom gave the impression that all his energy has been squeezed out of him.

On his third birthday the Taylor family organized a party. Irene placed Tom on the stool near her and started playing. Whenever she sat at the piano she enjoyed looking at Tom being all ears and eyes whatever his mother played.

She started playing "Happy Birthday to you", and other children sitting on the floor in the sitting room joined in the song.

The adults then went into the kitchen to have a celebratory drink away from the noise the children were creating. While in the kitchen they heard Happy Birthday song being played again.

'Who is still there?' asked Steve and looked around the table, while Irene went to check the sitting room.

She couldn't believe what she saw, rushed back to the kitchen and started whispering, gesticulating and pulling Steve toward the sitting room.

There was Tom, standing by the piano, playing the

same notes and even in the same key his mother played a while ago.

Irene was flabbergasted but her emotions were subdued when the children's parents started congratulating her on how well she thought Tom to play the song.

Irene liked to play for Tom a few of children's tunes before placing a sheet of music to play for her own pleasure. She used to give piano lessons before Tom arrived but observing her son sitting besides her she saw that Tom could concentrate deeper and for longer than any student she had.

'You see, he is not just normal. He may be an extra gifted child' said Steve and added 'In a year or two you could start giving him a couple of lessons a week but, mind you, without charge.'

Whenever Amanda went into Mathew's room she found him either reading, or writing into one of his computer files. This time she was curious seeing Mathew holding a very heavy book on his lap and at the same time making notes in his notebook.

'What are you reading sweetheart'.

'Oh just a book I borrowed from dad's study, it is very useful as I would like to learn, in a bit more detail, about the theory of chaos'.

After dinner when Mathew excused himself and went upstairs, Amanda said to her husband:

'Roger, I am worried about Mathew. Today I found him reading one of your books, he said it was to do with chaos or something like that'.

'Oh yes I bought that book because next year I might be giving a number of lectures on the subject. It is called "The theory of chaos" and is purely what it says.

Mathew is probably trying to impress me because I was a bit cold towards him the other day'.

'But Roger, Mathew is only nine and anyhow why don't you take him out at the weekend, fishing or walking. I think that he reads too much and is not developing physically. I am really worried about Mathew's health Roger'.

'He is really not made for any sport and detests any physical effort Amy. I have tried to encourage him but he simply refuses. Last week I gave him a book on mathematics teasers and asked him if we can do them together in the evening. He told me that he had done them last Saturday when he went to the library where he saw the same book.

I do not know how, but Mathew absorbs mathematics as if he has all the talents put solely into mathematics'.

'What do you mean by that Roger. Do you mean to say that Mathew can do only maths and nothing else?'

'No, not at all. Just that Mathew can learn anything, so far in mathematics, without any effort. Even my colleagues said that. In fact all of them said that. Last week when I collected him from the evening classes, I had to go back to the college and when he saw the blackboard full of symbols, I was teaching group theory earlier in the day, he already new that and much more. None of my colleagues said a word. They all stared in amazement. I asked him where did he learn this and he said that he read one of my books he found in my study. It took me two weeks to grasp the material from the book and I can say I read pretty fast'.

But Mathew did not feel that he had any special talent or talents. When he read a mathematics book, it was like watching an interesting film and remembering all the details.

Mathew did not miss his father's distancing himself but he thought to make an effort to please his mother who looked a bit sad lately. As his father was proud of his chess playing ability, Mathew decided to join the school chess club and learn to play chess.

He waited for the best time, during the dinner, to talk to his father.

'Dad, I joined the school chess club today, will you teach me how to play it?

'Of course Mathew, we could have an hour after

dinner and go through the rules, openings and have a few games. You are a bright boy, son, it wont take long for you to master it.'

Amanda was delighted in Mathew's interest in chess. She never learned to play it but for Mathew it would mean that he will be more involved with his schoolmates and maybe he and his dad will get a bit closer.

During the dinner both Amanda and Roger were involved in their separate thoughts. Amanda, as a mother, was pleased with Mathew and delighted at the prospect that Mathew and his dad could have something in common.

As for Roger, his thoughts were racing ahead to the time when he and Mathew could challenge each other in an occasional game, that is, if Mathew becomes sufficiently good. Roger played for the university when he was a student and now he plays for the University staff club and very seldom loses a game during the tournaments.

'You go upstairs Mathew and prepare the board and I will follow you in a minute.'

'Why don't you play here in the kitchen, and I will make you a nice cup of tea' said Amanda, hoping that she will be able to enjoy watching the two of them together.

'Yes Amy, that would be nice. Mathew you know where I keep the chessboard. If you bring it down now, we can start straight away.'

Roger was pleased how easy Mathew absorbed everything and the evening ended in delight for all the family.

'Dad, I would like to learn how to see what move is needed or what is best to do in a particular situation. Is there a book that I could get and read about it?'

'Of course Mathew, there are many books, some deal with beginnings of the game called openings and others go much deeper into the game and some deal with endings.

There are, as well, books that give complete games of famous players from tournaments around the world. There are a couple of books of mine on the shelf. You can start with them and if you need help, I am always available.'

Amanda was delighted and snuggled on the couch putting her head on Roger's shoulder and pretended to be watching the TV screen while dreaming of more good times to come to the Williams family. Mathew went upstairs switched on his computer and tried to go through the moves in chess his father explained to him.

It was easy to remember all the rules and even what move to play when your turn comes but to think of two, three or even more moves ahead, was not what he was able to do. His brain appeared to be reasoning in a way as if all possible moves are of equal importance and there was no point in analysing them all.

Mathew went to his father's study and took one of the chess books from the shelf.

'Today, we will spend an hour doing memory tests, said Mr. Aldridge, the teacher.

I will call out a group of numbers and you try to remember them and repeat them later when I ask you to. Now, there are different methods in storing information in the brain. One of them is to store the numbers in groups of two or three consecutive numbers and see them as pictures.

Some people have ability to remember faces or scenes while the others can remember numbers or sounds. To improve your memory, try to find out what you remember easiest and use that method to store in your brain any information you want to remember whether it is a set of numbers, a picture or a conversation you heard watching a film.'

'Excuse me Sir, are we allowed to write the numbers down?'

Not today Richard. This time we will test the memory of what we hear. The visual memory test will be next week.'

Richard Davenport was one of the best pupils in the

class but he had to work very hard to achieve that. He was very methodical for his age which he learned and absorbed from his parents. Everything in their house had to be in order including Richard's toys, which went back to their place as soon as he stopped using them. He never played with more than one toy at the time.

Mathew was bored with the way the teacher read out the random numbers and then asked the children in turn to repeat the sequence. For every set of numbers the teacher read Mathew, to amuse himself, converted the read numbers into the binary equivalent, and when his turn came he could not remember any.

At the end of the test Mathew was, with another two boys, at the bottom of the ability table.

A week later the teacher brought a bundle of sheets of paper and explained to the children the procedure of the visual test.

Then he gave each child a sheet of paper with the child's name on it as well as a set of seven numbers. The children were told to memorise the numbers and return the paper to him.

When Mathew's turn came to say what was on his piece of paper he said:

'First there was my name in the top left corner', ...and the whole class laughed aloud thinking that it was all Mathew remembered.

'Are you sure it was your name?' Asked Richard, and there was laughter again.

'Then there were seven numbers' and Mathew repeated all the seven numbers correctly.

New sheets were distributed with more numbers and at the end of the test Mathew was alone at the top of the list with seventeen digits set.

The teacher then took a blank sheet of paper and wrote down Mathew's name and under it an eighteen digit number and gave it to Mathew.

'Mathew, could you look at the set of numbers and give the paper back to me please?'

When asked to repeat the numbers, Mathew did that, correctly, without any hesitation.

Mr Aldridge went to the staff room and showed the test results to his colleagues.

'May be a freak result. You should repeat the visual test and compare the results to today's, said the headmaster after seeing Mathew Williams's results.

Mr Aldridge did just that and there were minor differences in the marks of the pupils in the class except for Mathew. His marks were as in the previous test, maximum points.

Mathew liked written examinations. He always wrote down the important details of any book he read and always cross-referenced the information he obtained from the book.

The 11+ exams was a special occasion for Mathew wanted to show his ability and create envy. He noticed through the last few years that more and more of his classmates looked upon him as if there was something not right with him. He new he was short and physically weak for his age but he didn't care because the only activities he cared for were mental ones.

Few months before the examinations Mathew started reading the exam questions of the previous ten years and their solutions as well as the books that were recommended.

When the exam date arrived, he simply sat down and started to put down, on the ruled notebook supplied, everything that was required. Mathew was a child with special love for mathematics. But not only maths. He could recollect any text, whether in numbers or letters if he saw it in written form.

It all came out when the 11+ exams results were published. Mathew achieved best results ever in the whole country and above his picture in a number of newspapers there was the name 'Mathew Einstein aged eleven' with the details of his marks.

His mother and father were interviewed and asked what type of food do they give him, his learning abilities, do they teach him at home, has he private tuitions and so on.

Mathew acquired a few extra friends, the ones who detested previously known bright boys and who were glad somebody "like them" surpassed the "elite".

But for Mathew there was no elation or feeling of achievement. In the class, he was compared to Spock in the TV space series. Mathew never laughed as if the word fun did not exist in his dictionary.

He wasn't spiteful either; he simply didn't care about others either in school or anywhere else.

'Mathew, what would you like as a present for the special achievement at the exams? Your father and I thought it would be nice for the three of us to go abroad on holidays, maybe somewhere warm and you and your father could do some fishing and swimming or just lazing about for a week or two'

'I would like, if that is not too much to ask, an in-ternet access so that even if I use it a lot, there would be a fixed charge. I would like that better than a holiday.' But if you and dad would like a holiday, why don't you go and Mrs Simpson, next door could look after me. She did say a while ago that she would be willing to look after me if you and dad need to go away. This would be a nice break for you and dad to be without me for a change.'

'No, we couldn't. You are not twelve yet.'

'I go to school on my own and do homework on my own and Mrs Simpson could cook for me for a week or two while you and dad are away.'

'Well, I will ask dad and see what he says.'

Mathew wanted so much to be able to explore, on the Internet, the reasons why he, Mathew, possessed such a good memory and yet he lacked ability in many other fields comparing to other boys in the school.

He was convinced that his body and mind were very different to all the boys in the school and yet he had no feelings of being superior or inferior.

He felt as if being placed among the beings very different from himself, even using different language, so that he, Mathew preferred to live his life in a self-isolation mentally and, wherever possible, physically too.

As his parents decided to go to Scotland for a week, his father organised the connection to the Internet to please Mathew.

Mathew, when his parents departed, gave Mrs Simpson the spare house key and she was delighted to leave him alone except when she brought him cooked lunch and dinner. She would look at Mathew and the computer, told Mathew to have a shower before going to bed, check that the house is locked and left, feeling sure that there is something not as it should be with that boy.

'Mum, there will be two school trips next term. One is a skiing trip to the French Alps and the other is a trip to Paris. I would like very much to go to Paris. It is for one week and we will be visiting all the museums and places of interest.'

'Of course you should go darling. Paris is such a beautiful city. Your father and I went there on our honeymoon, as you know, and I still remember all those wonderful places we visited. I'm sure you will enjoy it. In fact I have not stayed outside Lowestry since our trip to Paris not counting our trip to Scotland last year. We can go shopping soon and get you a rucksack. It will be much easier than carrying the suitcase.'

This was the first time that Mathew wanted to stay away from home and Amanda was secretly glad, because it would make him more outgoing and possibly divert him from his compulsive reading of mathematics books.

He was falling well behind physically for his age and Amanda worried every time Mathew showed a sign of a cold or any minor illness. The only things large on Mathew's body were his eyes and his genitals. In fact one could say much lager than normal.

'Roger, Mathew's school is organizing a trip to Paris. Isn't that fantastic? His first trip abroad and he goes to Paris where we went on our honeymoon.'

'There are a few places I would recommend ' said

Roger, 'such as the museum of Pure and Applied Mathematics. When your mum and I were there I could not visit it because it was closed for renovations.'

'Yes, I know about the museum. I already read about it, and there is another which covers the modern mathematics only. I hope I would be able to see both.'

'Why is it that whenever I try to pass on to Mathew some of my knowledge, he has already surpassed that, as if he can anticipate what I am going to say', said Roger to his wife when they were alone in front of the fire and Mathew was upstairs in his bedroom.

'Oh don't be angry Roger. This may be the turning point in Mathew's life I have been praying for. He might actually enjoy being with his friends outside school hours and he might even start going out after the Paris trip. He is now in grammar school and many of the schoolmates are new to him and there is a chance that Mathew might make few friends.'

'Well, let us hope so. Maybe we could go somewhere while Mathew is away. How about a trip to Vienna just for the two of us. You are a classical music fan and Vienna would give us a nice break. I think we deserve a holiday abroad after so many years without one.'

'Yes, I think it would be nice to be on our own once again and do things together as we used to.'

Roger managed to stop talking and just as well

because his thoughts would not have pleased Amanda. He had been in a strange mood lately. At times he wished they never had Mathew and were able to do things they enjoyed together for the nine years following their marriage. Then he would remember the first six years of Mathew's life and he was able to disperse those thoughts that depressed him.

But these thoughts surfaced with increased frequency, as Mathew got older. Not that he didn't want Mathew as his son. He did, but there was something that Mathew possessed or something that Mathew lacked, Roger wasn't sure what. Maybe he was imagining this but would it hurt Mathew if he took him to a psychologist.

Mathew showed very little affection for either of them and as time passed the distance between Mathew and his parents grew wider.

He never needed his father's or his mother's help with his homework and never wanted anybody to know what he was studying.

As he spent most of his time in the library or at home, in his bedroom, reading or writing, it was hard to do anything about it. If his mother came to his bedroom, he would continue to do what he was doing when she came in, and the visit never lasted long enough to start a proper conversation.

'Mathew what happened to the chess club you were to join at school?'

'We are doing fine. At the moment we are at the top of the five local schools table.'

'Are you playing in the team Mathew?' asked his dad.

'Yes I am. I play the first board.'

'What does it mean son?'

'It means that he is probably the best chess player in the class,' said Roger.

'You two can have a game then if Mathew is so good!'

'Yes, Mathew would you like a game. I would like to see how much you progressed since we tried the game, what, six months ago.'

Mathew brought the chessboard downstairs and selected to have black pieces.

Roger started with his King's Pawn Opening and the game started.

At the beginning Roger did not need to think much but he noticed that Mathew was responding without delay as well.

'It was very good Mathew, I thought you would not see that.'

'See what dad?'

'I almost took your knight.'

'Oh that' said Mathew and the game continued.

'Why did you play that move son, it will cost you a bishop?'

'That is all right, I can afford it.'

'Roger thought that Mathew needed a lesson of how to respect the opponent's strength and took Mathew's bishop with his pawn.

Mathew proceeded with a series of checks on Roger's king and soon the game was over.

'Mathew how did you do that. I have never seen that before?'

'I think it is called a Botvinik Variation or something like that. I am going to bed now, I have a headache. Good night.'

And that was the last game the two of them played.

'What is he like Roger?'

'My God he is a strange child Amy.

'But he must be gifted if he can beat you!'

'I really don't know. He beat me fair and square and didn't show any emotion.

I have never seen the moves he played yet from what I could see Mathew did not make a single mistake.'

'He certainly is,' thought Amanda and put her head on her husband's shoulder and decided not to think about that for now.

At the age of six when Tom started primary school, a year older than his schoolmates, he was by far the smallest among the twenty four boys and ten girls in his class.

It appeared that Tom could not concentrate and do the task he was asked to do but in fact he could be sitting in the class and play a tune or a classical piece of music, that he heard his mother play, in his head, while the teacher would be explaining a problem in maths or in science.

'Tom, what does eight times seven makes?'

'Tom Taylor!' The teacher would shout.

And the whole class would burst into a warm laugh as they were already used to Tom being absent minded during the class time.

Not a single praise was awarded to Tom at the end of the school term.

'Needs to concentrate, needs to work harder, has no interest in learning' and so on, the report stated at the end of the school year.

But Tom's parents were already carving a road on which he would soon travel.

They agreed for Tom to perform a half hour piano playing in their town hall and the agreed fee was more than Steve's three week's salary.

Steve was a sales representative for a well known life insurance company and was making good money. When he applied for the job they offered him a choice: a fixed salary and a small commission or no salary and a very attractive commission.

Steve chose the latter.

He was doing well for a few years and they decided to start a family. With time, Steve had to travel more and more in order to find new clients, lost interest in his work and often pretended not feeling well in order to stay at home.

Steve and Irene have already opened a bank account with joint names with Tom and were advised as to what was maximum time Tom was allowed, being underage, to work per month.

As a former music teacher, Irene has taken on to be Tom's manager and as she was familiar what and how Tom learned best, she always prepared Tom's program in advance.

Tom was only required to play what and when his mother decided.

For a while it was as if he was a famous film star and he would bow again and again on the stage and play with pleasure to the excited audience.

The audience loved Tom and his piano play. His small frame, dark hair, blue eyes and pale face made him look so vulnerable that anything he did, was followed with a warm applause.

It was like a fairy tale with Tom being the prince charming.

But within a couple of years of traveling and performing the enthusiasm disappeared and after an evening's performance Tom would feel completely exhausted and only wanted to go to bed and sleep.

'Tom, you should eat your dinner and then go to bed. There is another performance you are giving tomorrow,' his mother would say sitting opposite him in the hotel restaurant dining room.

'I am not hungry, I will have a big breakfast in the morning,' replied Tom and went to his bedroom.

'You see Steve, Tom doesn't have a singing voice and has a problem with sight reading, which means that he can not play by reading the notes without previous preparation. Actually the only way he can play is if I play first and he listens so his play is as good as he hears from me.'

'So, what are you trying to say Irene?'

'Well, Tom will be an attraction as long as he is young. After that he can learn new music by listening to a recording or to a live play.'

'Do you mean what I think you mean?'

'Yes I do. The money we are getting now will not be coming for ever.'

And Irene realized that what was troubling her was,

not so much her son's limited talent but his physical condition.

'Mathew, would you like to come to school on Saturday and have a few games of chess? We are forming the school chess team and I heard you were playing for your primary school team', asked David Bradshaw who was very keen to start the school chess club.

'OK', said Mathew, 'better being here than at home.'

After a few games with different schoolmates, Mathew was selected to play at number two board with David, as the captain, at number one board.

As Mathew felt no desire to compete with David for the number one board and David wanted so much to stay as the team captain, there was no animosity between the two.

David accepted Mathew as a good friend and Mathew felt that he can tolerate David and his chess club organizing activities because he, Mathew, will be away from his mum and dad for an extra half day a week.

David was sixteen and three years older that Mathew. His mother Margaret Bradshaw had him when she was a very young actress and David never new who his father was.

As David was growing up, his mother's career

improved and she traveled a lot, while David had to stay with his grandmother and later with the nanny.

At fifteen, David moved into the flat his mother bought for him and she visited him there whenever she could. Although they were apart most of the time, they were very close and David developed very pleasant personality.

He was very ambitious and even at the age of sixteen had already decided he would be a theatrical agent dealing with theatre and film stars.

'If we play like this, we will take the honours and be champions', said David after the first match the school chess club won against, what was considered to be, the strongest side in the league.

'Mathew would you like to come and have dinner at my flat next Saturday. Andrew Newman and Ian Robson will come as well. I don't cook so a takeaway will be on the table? I would like to discuss the tactics for our next match.'

The two boys, Andrew and Ian, were both sixteen and came from working class families. They were not brilliant students but hard working and enjoyed David's company.

'I would like that very much', said Mathew.

'Next Saturday at four it is then.'

Mathew would have preferred not to go but he

thought it might be better than being with his parents, when the library where he would have spent the day was closed.

He never mentioned David to his parents. Actually he never mentioned anything about the school, unless he was asked and even then the information he gave was very vague and scarce.

Mathew was the youngest and by far the smallest of the four boys in David's flat.

The boys laughed, told jokes and chatted about girls. Mathew pretended he was enjoying but actually he was bored and found the conversation a waste of time.

When he suggested a brainteaser, he was told not to mix school with pleasure so he started to think of a problem and then trying to solve it in his head.

'And you Mathew, have you ever done it?'

'Done what?' Sorry, I was thinking about something else.'

'Leave him alone. He is three years younger than you and has plenty of time to catch up with us'. Said David.

If Mathew was a bit taller, the teasing would not have stopped but, because of him being so small, they accepted David's words and left Mathew to his thoughts.

Paul and Anna were congratulating themselves for

being so far sighted and were proud of Joe and the way he progressed in the game of tennis.

'He never tires' said the tennis coach, Bert Langley, they hired to try and give Joe every opportunity.

'His tennis is good; in fact very good, but one thing he lacks is the ability to think and plan the game.

Joe doesn't see opponent's weak points and if told, when the game restarts he is back to his own game of hitting the ball across the net to the opponent's side of the court.'

'Could you do something to change his approach to the game?'

'I am not sure. I think he is ready to start as a professional but his overall ability will limit his success. Although Joe could earn sufficient amount to live comfortably, he will not get rich by playing tennis.'

'I don't believe that man,' said Anna. He was taking our money for the last two years and now he blames Joe.'

'Yes, maybe it would be better to see if we can find another coach to take over.'

But Joe wouldn't have it. He did not like mixing with people and Bert recognized it very early and kept Joe to himself and Joe was happy with that.

Bringing a new man to start afresh was something Joe did not want. So Anna and Paul signed a document for

Bert Langley to be Joe's coach for the period of five years from the date of him becoming a professional.

It was quite an expense the Browns spent on Joe and they were looking forward to have some of it coming back. But before that could happen, more money was needed to equip Joe and for hotel expenses.

Paul mentioned the prospect of his son becoming the professional tennis player to his colleagues at work and the firm Associated Chartered Accountants made Paul an offer to sponsor his son for a period of two years with one quarter of Joe's prize money going to the firm for the following two years.

'Now we can afford a holiday, just the two of us. What do you say to that Anna?'

'We can plan to be away for a week when Joe is at the training camp.'

'You know, if Joe could make it and win a few tournaments or even come near the top, prizes are so high nowadays, he can be financially better off than many brainy schoolmates of his.'

'I hope he does, Paul, I hope he does.'

'Mum, the teacher taking us to Paris said we shall need to get our passports for the trip. I thought that being in the European Union one could travel to France without the passport.'

'Not yet Mathew, they have not got that far yet.'

'How do I get the passport, mum?'

'Well, I think you need a photo taken, need a birth certificate and have to fill the passport application form.'

'And what do I do with all this?'

'Don't worry Mathew, dad and I will sort it out for you. This weekend we can go and get your photo taken and dad and I would do the rest.'

Mathew new he could rely on his mother to take care of such things and he forgot all about it until one morning when, he was at the gate, leaving his home on his way to school, the postman handed him a large envelope marked "The Passport Office".

Mathew was delighted but did not open it as there was the school bus coming and he placed the envelope into his schoolbag.

Mathew had school chess tournament that day, in the evening, and came home quite late.

'Mathew, we will have to go shopping to get you a ruck-sack and some clothes for your trip to Paris. How about Saturday?' asked his mum.

'Ah, yes, I completely forgot, my passport came today but I haven't opened the envelope yet.'

He went to get his schoolbag, opened it and took out the large envelope.

'Here it is mum, here is my passport.'

'Oh, and here is my birth certificate.'

Mathew looked at his birth certificate and felt there was something wrong with it. His name and date of birth were fine, but for the place of birth it said Hereditch. He knew where Hereditch was but that wasn't it.

And then it surfaced and he remembered.

'Mum it says here that I was born in Hereditch. Surely that must be wrong.'

'No Mathew, you were born in Hereditch, in a private hospital.'

'But, and Mathew's voice shook as he said, but I remember you told me once that you never left Lowestry since your honeymoon.'

Amanda suddenly got very pale, looked at Roger, looked back at Mathew and the words came out of her mouth full of fear:

'Mathew, sweetheart, dad and I would like to have a chat with you, could you sit here beside me on the couch, please.'

Suddenly Mathew felt he could not move. For the first time in his short life, he was thirteen last January; he felt insecure and did not know what was happening around him.

He obediently sat down beside his mother and immediately felt strange because they were going to tell him something he didn't want to hear. And his father's and his mother's words were like a murmur within a very loud noise.

Mathew was afraid to ask any questions aloud but inside his head he tried to solve the problem that had just occurred. But this problem was not like a maths problem where Mathew could use his brainpower and come up with the answer. It looked like a loop without an entry and without an exit.

'I was born in Hereditch but my mother wasn't there.' And Mathew could not continue to use his brain. The pain started first above and behind his eyes and then it spread to the back of his head. He felt as if he was going to vomit, tried to get up to go to the bathroom and then everything went black.

The next thing Mathew remembered, when he regained consciousness, was lying in his bed and his mum and dad sitting on the chairs beside the bed.

'Are you all right son?'

But Mathew did not answer and did not say a word. He stared at the ceiling and tried to remove from his brain the events that happened today.

Mathew never had a single dream, so all that he remembered was real, and he could not deal with it this time.

'Darling we started to tell you about your birth

certificate when you got very dizzy and had to carry you up here.'

Mathew recognized his dad's voice and yet he wasn't his dad, or was he?

'You just stay in bed son. The doctor is on his way. He will examine you and see if you need any medicine.'

'He must be here already I think I can hear the car in the drive. I'll go and bring him up.'

After examining Mathew, the doctor came downstairs where Roger and Amanda were waiting for him.

'Mathew is all confused and in a deep shock. I'm afraid it will take some time for him to be able to listen to the explanations about his genetic parents. You should have told him long time ago about the adoption and anything else you knew about his parents and reasons for him being given for adoption.'

'Yes, we should have, but every time we thought of telling him, we found a reason to delay and this is the result.'

Roger did not speak but his face showed anger.

'We have always done everything we could for Mathew and now his behaviour is as if we are strangers to him.'

'But you are! At least that is how he sees you today. And it may take some time for him to accept the news of him being adopted and the rest. I think you should wait for Mathew to feel the need for answers and then you better tell him all he wants to know,' said doctor Hearn, 'and please do not hesitate to call me if the need should arise.'

Amanda went upstairs a few times that evening and placed food and medicine on Mathew's bedside table but every time she came Mathew pretended to be asleep, or at least Amanda thought so.

When she went up to his room the next morning to see if there was any change, she found the room empty.

At first she thought Mathew was in the bathroom but when she saw the bathroom door open, she called: 'Roger!' and then the panic started.

'Mathew has no friends really and never stayed away from home before.'

'And he even left his set of house keys', said Amanda when she instinctively went to the front door.

'What shall we do Roger?'

'Well, we have to wait for the school to start and then you can phone the school secretary and ask if Mathew has arrived or, you go to school and say that Mathew forgot his sandwiches or something like that.'

'Yes, but what if he is not there?'

'You can find an excuse, can you not, I have meetings all day and can not get out of any even if I wanted to'

'Roger, it is our son we are talking about.'

'I am not sure any more. It feels as if we never had a son to start with.'

Amanda was falling to pieces and couldn't help the situation herself. Why could they not be a normal happy family?

'I don't want to listen to any more music today mum. I feel tired and have a headache.'

'OK Tom, you go and have a rest and we can continue in the afternoon.'

'Why don't you teach him to read the music himself Irene?'

'You know, Steve, I am almost sure he can not learn that skill.'

'Rubbish, every musician reads the music. Some are better than others but they can all read the notes. How else can they learn all that by heart?'

'Exactly. They all can by looking at the notes, except Tom. He can memorise the music only through his ears.'

'Maybe you haven't tried hard enough to teach him to do a bit of work for himself.

He just sits there with his eyes closed and you have to play and play.'

'Oh leave me alone. Nag, nag, nag; that is all I get from you. You don't see this as work, do you? Well let me tell you something Steve: Tom and I are working very hard while you live like a parasite. No wonder Tom is tired. Actually both Tom and I are exhausted and I don't know how long we can go on without a break?'

Tom was still at the bottom of the stairs going up when the argument started and he stopped and listened.

'So now it is all my fault isn't it?'

'Please yourself Steve. I'm going out.'

Tom rushed up the stairs and just as he reached the landing, his mother came out from the music room, put on her coat and went out.

Tom locked himself in his bedroom and when his father came and knocked on the door, he pretended to be asleep.

He was dreaming. The sun was shining and he was in the field lying on the warm grass and the clouds were a stage where the music was being played and he, Tom, was just listening and not requiring to remember in order to reproduce it later.

There was a warm applause and an encore that grew lauder and lauder.

It made Tom wake up but the applause was still there until he realised that it was the knocking on his bedroom door. Tom got up to open the door and there was his mother.

'David, it is me, Mathew, may I come up please?'

'Of course Mathew, push the door when you hear the buzzer!' and David pressed the buzzer button, letting Mathew into the building.

While Mathew climbed to the third floor where David's flat was, David tried to think of a reason why Mathew called at this time of day.

'I'm sorry to wake you up David but I had nowhere else to go.'

'It's no trouble Mathew. I always get up early to do my exercises, but tell me what happened?'

'I am really not sure David. When my passport came yesterday, there was my birth certificate. It said that I was born in Hereditch yet my mum told me some time ago that she had never been outside Lowestry since their honeymoon. When I asked them about it they told me I was adopted.'

'Many children are adopted Mathew. It is not the end of the world you know.'

'You see David I always thought there was something wrong with me. Now I am almost sure there is, and I wonder what my real parents were really like.'

'Like what?'

'Like my size. I have always been the smallest in the class yet I am almost a year older than any of the boys or even girls. Then look at my memory. When I see something written, it is as if there was a photograph placed in my brain.'

'But look how good you are at chess. I think you are even better than me.'

'No David, I can play chess because I am able to memorise so much. You see, when I play chess, I look at the positions of the pieces on the board and compare this to one of the games by famous chess players I know by heart. Then I know what move to make. But I have not slept at all last night and I am very tired. Could you let me stay here till you come back from school?'

'Of course you can stay Mathew but what if anybody asks questions? What shall I say?'

'Could you say that you didn't see me, just for today, please?'

'OK Mathew but only for today.'

'Anna don't forget we have to give one quarter of Joe's earnings to my firm.'

'I know, and after taking all expenses into account we have made a net profit of forty two thousand pounds.'

'Do we have to pay tax on that?'

No Paul, that is not our money but Joe's, and I think that half of it should be put into his investment account.'

'And what happened with the sponsors. Have they contacted you?'

'Yes they have and that will be over and above Joe's earnings from playing.'

'Joe looks great in the photographs they are going to use; I just wish he would smile now and then. Remember him as a two year old? Even then he seldom gave a smile.

How odd nature can be? Such a nice body, full of energy and yet his IQ is so low that I can not stop worrying about him.'

'Maybe Bert Langley was right when he told us he believed Joe would not improve. You know, this might be his limit. If so, we have to do our best for Joe to have his future finances settled as soon as possible.'

'I agree. Instead of saving I think we should invest for his pension.

'Paul, do you think we should tell Joe everything about his birth or is it better to leave it for a while?'

'He is so serious about being professional player; I think we better leave it for a while.'

But nothing could upset Joe. He played like a robot whether practicing or in a tournament, giving everything his body could supply and never tiring.

This endless source of energy resulted, quite often,

in demands to test Joe for any possible use of banned substances, but he was always clear.

Now and then, when an opponent saw Joe's way of returning the ball, Joe would have quite a fight to win by making the opponent tired.

Bert new what tournaments to enter Joe to produce results and Paul and Anna had to admit that it was the right decision to keep Bert Langley as Joe's coach.

Mathew stayed at David's flat for the night and when they arrived to school together, the following day, the headmaster asked Mathew to come to his office.

There, to his surprise, were his parents.

'Take a seat Mathew', said the headmaster.

'Hello Mathew! Said Amanda in a soft voice; your dad and I would like to talk to you. Will you let us please?'

'I don't know who my dad is, but I intend to find out. And my mother as well.'

'Mathew, we are sorry, we should have explained to you about your adoption but we tried to do what we thought was best for you. In fact we know very little. We were on a waiting list for the adoption for about two years and one day, out of the blue, we got a phone call to come to the hospital to see a young baby whose mother died. When we saw you, you were very week and only two weeks old. Your dad and me decided there and then to take you as our child. No other information was given to us.'

Mathew did not show any emotion but the little colour there was on his face had vanished and he just stared straight ahead.

'Mathew' said the head, 'you are still very young and, for all that has happened, very upset so let me put forward a proposal: You stay with your parents, or if you want, with Mr and Mrs Williams, and take your time to find out whatever you can and want about your genetic parents. I will give you an approved leave from school for as long as it takes you to sort yourself out.

When you think that you have done all you could, we will meet again here and have another talk. What do you say to that?'

Mathew did not answer but stared in front of him without even a single expression.

'Mathew, please, you will have complete privacy and we will talk to you only if you want us to?'

'I will be there tonight, after the chess competition', said Mathew, got up and left the head's office without further word.

Amanda excused herself and went to the ladies. She could not hold her tears any more.

'Tom, could you come downstairs please!' said Irene

as Tom opened his bedroom door. Tom noticed tears in her eyes and her voice trembling.

'Is everything all right mum?' asked Tom as he entered the music room and saw his mother using her handkerchief to wipe her eyes.

'Tom, your father and I had an argument.'

'I know mum, I heard you before you went out.'

'He left me a note saying he's had enough of you and me and we can do whatever we want. Tom, dad will not be coming back.'

'I'm sorry mum, maybe if I had more brains, he would not have gone.'

'No Tom, you are a nice boy and have a lot of talent and we will carry on, just the two of us.

Tom sat beside his mother, gave her a warm hug and the two of them cried together in silence.

Maybe we could have a holiday abroad for a week, what do you say? I will cancel your next performance; I'll say you have a flu and we'll go to the sun.'

'That would be nice mum, just the two of us.'

Tom was very pleased about the week's holidays not because of going abroad but because he would be free from listening to the piano music and from playing. Lately, whenever he had to listen for a long spell, his head would start aching and he could not hear the notes as well as he did when his head was light and fresh.

A week's holiday was the best thing that could have happened to Tom and his mum.

Tom had no headache for the whole week and Irene completely forgot they were going to be alone from then on.

'Ill be away all day today', said Mathew to Amanda as he walked towards the front door. He made a couple of sandwiches, took an apple and a small bottle of water, put everything into his rucksack and checked that he had his passport and his birth certificate with him.

He was on his way to start the quest to discover what and why all this happened to him. Who were his parents and why did his parents abandon him?

The birth certificate had a place of birth: Hereditch, Hereford and that was his destination at the start of the search.

Mathew got an early bus out of Lowestry and traveled to Shrewsbury. He was lucky and got a connection bus bound for Birmingham, which would take him straight to Hereditch, just outside Birmingham.

There was a stewardess on the bus to Birmingham taking orders from passengers for sandwiches and teas. When she came to Mathew she said:

'Are you all right? You look very pale.'

'Yes, I am fine', replied Mathew.

'There is a bag in the pocket in front of you if you need one.'

'Thank you I am fine.'

'There is a young boy upstairs', said the stewardess to the coach driver. 'He is so pale it looks as if he may not last the journey. I think I will keep an eye on him.'

The journey was to take just over three hours and Mathew tried to have a rest but his brain was so active that when the bus finally arrived at Hereditch coach station, he was very tired.

The birth certificate he carried with him, stated that it was issued by the Registry Office, Hereditch and he proceeded to the Town Hall where the Registry Office was located.

Mathew followed the sign Registry Office and when he reached it, there was a lady behind the window.

'Yes, what can I do for you young man?'

'This is my birth certificate. My mother died when I was born and I was adopted. Could you tell me what I need to do to find a bit more about my birth mother and my birth father?'

'Yes I can. Your adopted parents can request some details about your birth parents any time they want but, I am afraid, you can not do that until you are eighteen.'

'I have come all the way from Lowestry. Could you

at least give me the name of the cemetery where my birth mother was buried please?'

'I am afraid I cannot. The law is very strict here, but your adopted parents can get that information if they ask for it. I am very sorry.'

'Thank you very much. You were very helpful.'

And that was all Mathew could do in Hereditch.

By then he was so tired that he simply bought a sandwich and took the first bus back to Shrewsbury. By the time he caught a bus to Lowestry and walked home it was past ten in the evening. Roger and Amanda were in the sitting room but scared to say anything.

'I couldn't get anything in Hereditch this time and I am very tired. I will tell you the rest in the morning.'

Next morning Mathew waited for his father to leave before he came downstairs.

His mother was full of fear and apprehension as she waited for Mathew to start the conversion.

'I went to the Registry Office in Hereditch, but was told that I could get the information about my birth parents when I reach my eighteenth birthday. Could you tell me what you know please?'

'Mathew dear, as I said in your school the other day, your dad and I, or if you prefer, Roger and I were on a waiting list for an adoption, as I couldn't conceive, for about three years, when suddenly a call came one evening from the adoption agency to go to the South Birmingham Private Clinic where there is a baby available for adoption.

We drove the next morning to Hereditch and the officer from the adoption agency took us to the maternity ward to see the baby. We were told that the father died soon after the baby was conceived and that the mother died at birth.

We had to decide there and then and, after seeing you, we said yes. That was all we were told and two weeks later all the paperwork was ready and we went to bring you home, I mean here, which was your home till now.'

'I would be very grateful if you could do something else for me. Could you contact the Adopted Children Register which is in Southport, and apply for the Standard Certificate of birth for me.'

'Of course Mathew, I will go tomorrow to the Council Offices here in town and ask for the application form and post it straight away. The council offices are closed on Mondays.'

A week later a letter arrived from the Adopted Children Register with Mathew's birth certificate. Mathew hurriedly opened the envelope and reading the document said:

'This is not the right certificate. It is called the Adoption

Certificate, and I wanted the Standard Certificate of my birth.' And with these words he went upstairs.

Mathew decided to obtain the Standard Birth Certificate himself. He went to the Council Offices and found the appropriate application form CA14 to obtain his certificate of birth at the Family Record Centre in Southport.

But then, when he read the booklets ACR99 andACR100, the disappointment came as he realised that he needed to be eighteen before he could start the search for his birth parents, just as the lady in the Hereditch Registry Office had told him.

Mathew now knew that he was adopted and that he could not have inherited any genes from what he thought were his parents.

He felt desperate but powerless to do anything as all the booklets he obtained from the Registry Offices stated that he must reach the age of eighteen before starting any search.

This realization made him very depressed.

'I have to wait for two years just to find out where my mother is buried. What were my name and my surname? Were my parents normal people or did I inherit any genes that made me the way I am?'

Mathew hated the house he lived in and everything surrounding him there. He wished he could be on his own and that he could wake up and be eighteen years old.

Mathew spent almost all his time in his room except when there were chess competitions. He avoided going to school as much as possible. The school head and Amanda had many discussions as to what to do but to no avail.

Mathew did not study and it was obvious that he will not pass his GCSE exams. David was the only person in whom Mathew would confide and every now and then Mathew would spend a night at David's flat. David was amazed how much detail Mathew could remember and one evening, while the two of them were watching an old film, said:

'You know, Mathew, your memory is so good you should make money using it.'

'David, who would pay me for remembering all the chess moves I have in my head?'

'I'm not talking about the chess. Say you enter for a quiz competition where you have to know a lot about a particular subject, book or a film or even about the events in history. You could memorise in advance and win with ease any of the competitions we see on the box.'

'I suppose I could. But what would that do for me?'

'Well, if you have money, you are independent and can live anywhere you desire.'

Mathew did not answer but his brain went into top

gear and raced through all the possibilities he could think of.

'You have something there, David, I will think about that.'

The next morning when David got up he noticed Mathew looked unusually pale and quiet.

'You look ill, Mathew, can I do anything for you before I leave?'

'Not a thing, David. I didn't sleep well last night. I was busy thinking about the advice you gave me and I think I can do something but I don't want to be on TV. Maybe I can organize a show on my own here in Shrewsbury.'

'What show are you talking about? Asked David still half asleep and not ready to receive complicated statements.

Mathew tried to explain his idea about how to become independent and be able to live on his own but David did not absorb a thing.

'Joe, let us sit down and talk for a while', said Bert and took the racket from Joe's hand.

'Yes Mr Langley', replied Joe and did what he was asked to do.

Joe was almost twice the size of his coach but he

never questioned his coach and always tried to do what was asked of him.

Bert Langley could not understand how a young boy like Joe, with the physical ability he possesses, could not use it to his advantage.

'I think you are using too much of your energy and not enough of your brains when you hit the ball.'

'What should I do then Mr Langley?'

Bert put a large notebook on his lap and drew an outline of the tennis court.

'You see Joe: you are here, on the touchline and your opponent has returned the ball and stayed at the side of the court. What should you do?'

'I'll do whatever you tell me, Mr Langley!' I always try to do that.'

'I know Joe, I know.'

Bert Langley was delighted when he was asked two years ago if he would like to be Joe's coach. Joe was twelve then, blond bushy hair and blue eyes, made Bert imagine that he saw a new world champion in not too distant future.

Joe could hit the ball, he could run, and he had stamina of an athlete in full training.

But he soon noticed that Joe always returned the ball along the court. Bert tried to make Joe see that and told Joe:

'Joe, hit the ball so that it lands away from your opponent.'

'But which side Mr Langley?'

'Well, if your opponent is here', and Bert made a cross on the court drawing, ' you should place your shot there.'

'Yes Mr Langley, I'll do that next time.'

'OK Joe, I'll switch on the gun to assimilate the service and you try to return the serve, once to the left and once to the right.'

'Yes Mr Langley.'

But Joe, for some reason did not do that.' All the returns were back along the court length. If the gun served to the centre part of the serving area, Joe returned the ball to the centre of the opponent's court, and if the gun served to the side, Joe returned the ball along that sideline.

'OK Joe. I'll switch off the service gun. Let us try something else now.

'You will play alone on this side, against Bob and me, on the opposite side. I will serve and you have to return the ball once to me and once to Bob. Is that clear?'

'Yes Mr Langley, I am ready!'

Bert served half a dozen balls to near the center line and Joe returned all the serves back along the centre line.

'Joe, I served about a dozen times and you returned all the balls to me!'

'Yes Mr Langley.'

'But I asked you to return the ball…

OK Joe. We will stop and you take the rest of the day off.'

'You see Bob', said Bert when Joe left, 'there is something with this boy that puzzles me. He has all the physical abilities required to become an excellent tennis player and yet he plays like that gun over there, he hits the ball in one direction only, parallel to the length of the court.. I feel I will never be able to change that.'

'He is still young Bert. One day he could just click and start using his brain.'

'If he has one. Sometimes I wonder whether there is any of it in there.'

'He is fourteen Bert isn't he. Some boys still suck their thumbs at his age. Give him time and he will change.'

'Yes young man, what can I do for you?'

'Thank you for seeing me Mr martin. I. . .'

'Wait a minute, I have seen you somewhere before but could not put my finger to it.'

'You might have seen my picture in the papers a few years ago.'

'My God, it is you isn't it?

Yes, I remember you. They used to call you Einstein then, didn't they?

Have a seat young man. You have not changed since I saw your pictures in the papers two or three years ago.'

'I see you remember my 11+ exams Mr Martin. I came here to make you a proposal for a family show and, at the same time, to make a nice sum of money for you and me, that's if you are interested.'

Young man, I have many actors, acrobats and agents and I can go down the alphabet and everywhere there are people trying to get a break. It would need to be something extra special for me to bite, if you see what I mean.'

Mr Martin kept his hall in excellent condition and turned down many proposals before but this young boy, in fact he looked like a child, with dark hair, blue eyes and the face that looked as if it never saw the sunlight, fascinated him and he decided to give him a few minutes of his time of which he had a lot lately.

He and his wife decided to leave the rat race and work only enough to live in moderate comfort. They had no children of their own and have made good provisions for themselves.

'I have prepared everything written but let me present you with my idea of the show.

You organise your hall, I believe it has a capacity of

about 2000 seats, for a family show and advertise my performance where 50% of profits goes to a number of charities, selected by the audience.

There would be an entry fee of course.

Each head of the family in the audience gives me, upon entry, their seat number, name and surname, their partner's name and surname, ages or dates of birth, their birth places, number of children and their names and let us say where they, their wives and possibly their children, work or go to school.

All this information will be written with an extra copy.

After I read the details, the head of the family gets back the original and, a copy is put into a filing cabinet witnessed by the panel selected by the audience.

After that my show starts. I invite any person from the audience to ask me to reveal any of the above for any member of the audience giving me the seat number or any other data on the ticket.

Now, if my answer is correct, that person pays £10, and if my answer is incorrect, that person receives £10. I could even bargain with the invited person for higher stakes if he or she feels that it is worth to risk more money. Whoever pays the money, decides what charity the proportion of it goes to.

There could be a comedian or two if you want but

I think these are main points and I believe it should be very profitable.'

There was a long silence. Mr Martin kept his eyes closed as if he was in a deep sleep.

Actually he was calculating the number of questions assuming the hall is half full, and

came out with a figure of about fifteen thousand.

'Young man, have you thought of the possibility that you get stuck and it would make me bankrupt?' There are over fifteen thousand questions in what you propose.'

'Well', said Mathew, 'why don't you test me. You give me fifteen thousand words, number each word from one to fifteen thousand and then test me. I need only half an hour to look at the text.'

'You are serious about it aren't you', said Mr Martin.

'Yes I am. I have a few thousand pounds and I can deposit the cash with you to give you security for the first show, in case you think I may not be able to answer the questions put forward.

By then I am sure you will be convinced. 'You can have all the profits from the bar and the rest and 15% of the takings.

'I will claim expenses of about five thousand pounds and from the rest I'll give 50% to the charities selected. If you want this type of a show, a family show, here is my mobile number. I am always available. Thank you very much for your time Mr Martin.'

Mathew offered his hand to say good buy and left.

For the first time in his life Mathew felt elated. If his proposal was accepted he, Mathew, would be able to have his own place and forget about his adopted parents

Geoff Martin, on the other hand, was flabbergasted. He never saw anybody with such confidence especially somebody of that age. He left his office and called his wife to join him for lunch.

'Maura what would you think of me if I, sort of, rent the hall to a child nicknamed Einstein. You remember the eleven plus genius of a few years ago, the little boy that looked like a child. He came to me and proposed to run a charity show. Well, sort of charity as, to use his words, he and I would make quite a bit of money as well. I think I will give him a test.'

'What are you talking about Geoff, what sort of a test?'

'Well he claims he can remember up to fifteen thousand numbers or names by seeing the lot just once. I think that if he can do that we may not be selling the hall yet after all.'

'But I thought we decided to take it easy Geoff and this would keep you very busy!'

'Not so busy Maura, one show a week would be just

right and anyhow if the boy is what he says he is, I would really enjoy it.'

Geoff Martin then explained to his wife the conversation he had with the "Einstein boy".

'You know, there is something about him that I admire but at the same time I am scared to even think of what goes on in his head.'

'So why are you telling me all that. Do you want me to decide for you?'

'Your sister's daughter Beth is going out with that young man Allen. Isn't he some sort of a computer expert?'

'He is and I believe a very ambitious one at that.'

'If so, he could probably create a random list of fifteen thousand numbered words and we can see what would be the outcome?'

'Why are you not giving the opportunity to Allen instead of to somebody you don't even know?'

'Maura, when have my instincts deserted me? Throughout my whole career in this business I have never been more enthusiastic than now.'

'Mr Langley, what did I do wrong today?'

'Joe you are a good boy and you are trying very hard. Maybe it would be good to take a break from tennis for a couple of weeks. I'll try to arrange a talk with your parents as soon as I can. You go and change and then sit and watch your friends and observe what they do in their games.'

'Would it be all right if I go home instead Mr Langley?'

'Of course it would Joe. You have played a lot of tennis in the last month or so.'

Joe was not tired. Physically he was never tired as if there was an enormous amount of energy inside him, but his mental state made him look as if he lacked energy.

When Joe came home, the house was empty and he went straight to bed and fell into a deep sleep.

Paul and Ann were visiting friends. Paul's colleague Ian McLintock and his wife Liz were celebrating their first grandson's birth and many of Ian's friends from the Associated Chartered Accountants came including Paul with his wife Ann.

'It was a good move to sponsor your son Paul. The firm has already got their money back with interest so he must be doing well in tennis.'

'Not too bad although there were expenses to be paid we never thought would arise but at least Joe is doing fine.'

'He is taller than you now, isn't he Paul?'

'Yes, he is.'

At that moment Ann came and asked Paul if she can

have a word. As they moved away from the others she said:

'Paul, I have tried to get Joe at home but there was no answer. I thought he was coming home early today.'

'He is probably enjoying himself at the club. Anyhow we will be going home soon too.'

But when they came home the house was in the dark.

'Paul he is still not home. Shall I try the club and see if he is still there.'

'Do if you want to.'

When she dialed the number the voice came on:

'Bert Langley!'

'Mr Langley, is Joe there please?'

' Hallo Mrs Brown, Joe went home about three o'clock, at least that was where he said he was going to.'

'Thank you very much, good night Mr Langley.'

At that moment Joe appeared at the sitting room door.

'Hey guys, did you enjoy yourselves?'

'Joe, I was worried, I thought you were still out.'

'No, I felt a bit bored and fell asleep in my room.'

'Mum, I think Mr Langley wants to talk to you about having a break for a week or two. Maybe we can go somewhere warm and sunny.'

'Of course Joe. This is first time ever that you mention a holiday. We'll certainly do that.'

'Paul I think we had been neglecting Joe's needs in the past. Would you be able to take couple of weeks off work and the three of us could just laze about in the sun?'

'Not at this time of year Ann, this is our busiest period. You and Joe go and have a nice rest. You both deserve it.'

Geoff Martin obtained a dictionary words from Microsoft word processor with a number attached to each word selected at random.

He had the printout on his desk when Mathew came in.

'Mathew, here is the material I have for your memory test as you call it. When would you like to start?'

'We can start now if that is all right with you Mr Martin?'

'Wright then. It is now ten o'clock. At eleven o'clock I'll take the bundle from you and will ask you about fifty questions. That should be enough for me. Where do you want to read the material Mathew?'

'I'll sit there on the sofa and will come back when I am finished.'

After just fifty minutes, Mathew got up and said he was ready.

'My God son, I wouldn't be half way yet even just reading and you say you memorised all of it. I want to see that.

There were thirty four pages with four columns and about forty lines in each column containing a word and a random number preceding the word. Each line contained about four words with a number attached to it.

Goeff Martin selected a word at random from page one and Mathew gave correct number allocated to the word. After twenty pages he gave Mathew a number and the young man replied with the word associated with the number in question.

After forty questions Geoff Martin stopped, saying:

'Mathew, I don't know how you do it but I am more than convinced. Leave it with me for now and I'll give you a call in a few days.

Two days later Mathew's phone rang and as it was a new number that he did not recognize, he said:

'Yes!'

'This is Geoff Martin. Is that Mathew?'

'Yes Mr Martin, nice to hear from you!'

'Mathew could you come to see me sometime this week. I have prepared an agreement, based on your proposal and, if you agree the terms, we could sign it and the show could start anytime you are ready. What do you say Mathew?'

'I'm speechless Mr Martin. And I'm delighted. Would tomorrow morning be all right with you?'

'Tomorrow is fine. I'll see you at about ten Mathew.'

Mathew tried to call David to tell him about the show but the answer phone said he was out, so Mathew decided to look for a place to live after he received the first pay from the show he, Mathew, was going to have.

'Well Mathew, what do you say; is it all right with you?'

Couldn't be better Mr Martin. Let us sign the papers and see about the opening day.

'Mathew, are you sure you have enough material for the show. Suppose the questions don't come up to a number you have planned?

'I thought about that too. I studied a book on how the politicians and people like that make audience want to ask questions by appearing vulnerable. I could point out how many wives are older than their husbands, how many men are called Martin and play with the letters and numbers of the details they would give me to start with. All that should entice the audience to respond. I am sure of that.'

'And you will be able to remember all these things by just having a glance at them?'

'That won't be difficult, but if you would like me to do anything else, I can include that as well.'

'I don't know Mathew. My wife says I must be mad going to do this but I am so excited, it feels like starting all over again. I will organize everything around the show and it is up to you what you do during the show itself.'

'I'm sure you won't be disappointed and as you do all the bookkeeping, could you do my accounts as well, for a fee of course.'

'Say we start the following Saturday. Would that give you enough time to prepare yourself?'

'We have a date. Thank you Mr Martin for trusting me.'

'Oh one more thing Mathew. I have asked my solicitor about employing you as a minor and his answer was that it is legal providing you do not work more than eight hours a week. So I wont be breaking any laws.'

The show started well and after three weeks the Hall was always almost full.

Mathew found a place of his own and his adopted parents agreed for him to move wanting to choose the option of minimum damage.

Geoff Martin enjoyed seeing his star and the only performer of the show resting, prior to his appearing on the stage, in a little room at the back where there was a name Mathew written on the door with a large star above the name.

Mathew would open a tin of fruit, pour the contents

into a bowl and add a large amount of fresh cream and that was his treat after every show.

On one such occasion when Mathew was just finishing his bowl of fruit he was surprised by a knock on his stage room door.

'Hello, may I come in?' and she entered and sat in front of Mathew's desk.

'My name is Claire, Claire Battersby. I attended a few of your shows and am still fascinated by your ability to do all those things.'

Claire was a smallish girl although much taller than Mathew with a nice but slim body and short hair. She was sent to try and obtain from Mathew his secret trick. At least that was what Allen Randall believed to be.

A trick, to impose a belief upon the audience that it was possible to memorise so much data and retrieve it afterwards, as the computer dictionary calls it Random Access Memory or RAM.

Allen created a random selection of fifteen thousand words numbered from one to fifteen thousand and alternatively, he used a text from a book and used a set of randomly selected numbers from one to fifteen thousand for his girlfriends uncle. Later he was told that the boy, Mathew Williams, after just reading the lot only once, did manage to come up with the correct word for any given number out of fifteen thousand.

Allen Randall was sure that no human was able to have such a memory and if he could find out the way Mathew Williams did it he, Allen Randal, would do it even better.

Mathew was not enjoying the conversation with this girl. Her presence made him feel somewhat uneasy. Yet, he could not send her away. He was fascinated by this girl sitting in front of him, although he could not imagine why.

First, why did she pretend she was at many of his shows when she only attended one, and second, being close to her, he felt a sensation never before experienced?

His groins were in a state that he could not explain.

'Maybe I need to go to the loo', Mathew thought, and yet he felt no urgency at all.

'So, what did you want to talk about? You said on the phone it wasn't going to take more than a few minutes.'

'At the show you were coming up with the answers as if you were reading them rather than remembering them. How was it possible?'

'Some people can remember more than others. I am one of those with better memory, in fact better than anyone I know. You can remember some things and with practice you can improve, but you need to have a lot in you to start with.'

'When did you notice you were so good in remembering?'

'Ah, ever since I could remember if I may use the expression.'

'You must be very clever and talented.'

'Don't call it talent. It is the ability of power of mind to take in any information and then to release it at will.'

Claire tried to remember these words to be able to tell Allen about the power of mind.

'Have you ever seen me before?' Asked Claire just to see if he could get confused and reveal anything else that she may pass on to Allen.

'Yes, as a matter of fact you were at the show last Saturday, sitting in row 17, seat I believe 26, with your brother Allen Randall and his girlfriend.'

'My God, so when I introduced myself, you already new who I was?'

'Of course I did, I even know that your birthday is next week and you will be 22. What I don't know is why your and your brother's surnames are not the same if you are brother and sister.

'My God, and for how long do you retain all that information?'

'Well, most of it I remember for a very long time if I think it is important.'

Claire always felt she needed to have a safe distance

in conversation with other people but with Mathew she felt quite at ease, as if the two of them had something in common.

'As you know so much about me, would you like to have dinner with me on my birthday?'

Mathew heard himself saying: 'Yes that would be nice,' and immediately regretted it.

Yet he did not try to change his answer. Maybe because nobody showed interest in him for as long as Claire did although in his mind there was a question: Why?

Claire put forward her hand and said: 'Great, till next week, and please call me Claire and may I call you Mathew?'

'Of course you may.'

'Here is my mobile number. Wednesday or Thursday would be fine with me.'

Claire enjoyed having sex with Allen although he always had to be in charge and was very selfish and never considered how she felt. It was always quickly in and quickly out of bed for him.

This thing that he wanted from her, to find out about Mathew, was hurting her but Claire never complained to Allen. She did not love Allen. She did enjoy his body and did not want him to distance himself from her. And she was not jealous of his real girlfriend.

When she told Allen what she learnt, Allen just said: 'You must do better than that!'

And that was that. That hurt Claire and she decided to end their relationship there and then.

On the afternoon of Claire's birthday Mathew called and suggested a meeting near a small restaurant he occasionally visited but when they met, Claire said:

'I went to bring a takeaway for two and put it in the oven. I recall, from your show, that you said you did not like eating in restaurants. So if you would like we can eat at my place.'

'You see, your memory is not bad either, and yes, I would prefer to eat at your place, the less people around me the better.'

Claire had her place very tidy but it was the kitchen, the dining room and the bedroom all in one, with a little entry hall and the bathroom.

'Welcome to my palace Mathew, I hope you will like the meal. As Mathew was taking off his coat, Claire went to the kitchen part of the room and took a bottle of wine from the fridge. We will have this with our meal but first to toast my birthday will you try a small schnapps.'

'A small what?'

'It is a continental drink, made from fruit or something like that and is quite strong.'

'Is that why the glasses are so small?'

'Yes, and you are supposed to down it in one go.'

Mathew had an occasional drink in the last few years but he never enjoyed more than a few sips of beer.

He did as Claire instructed and as soon as the liquid passed his throat, he felt very warm all over and again the strange sensation came to his groin.

'Your face is quite red, it shows you never had schnapps before.'

'You are right there' said Mathew feeling very hot indeed.

'Would you like a bit more of this schnapps?'

'No thanks, one is more than enough, I feel as if I am on fire.'

Claire was now standing beside Mathew. She was much taller than him and even Mathew's body looked weaker than hers.

'Take your tie off, and you'll feel better. Sit down on the bed and I'll do it for y….

'What is that in your trousers Mathew?'

Claire asked as her hand accidentally touched his groin.

'Oh, my God Mathew, you are…. and she put her hand there again.

Mathew could not move. His eyes followed Claire's hands but his body felt as if it was frozen in a very hot ice, frozen but burning. But the burning did not cause any pain. On the contrary, and it was a sensation that

Mathew could not describe as he had never been in such a state before.

'Oh God, Mathew, oh God Mathew!'

Mathew never even kissed a girl before. He never experienced such a sensation.

'Oh God, Mathew!.

Claire was an honest girl with her own morals which might have not been the recognized in a normal society but she never took advantage of anybody. She did not think, being with Mathew, was doing anything wrong.

She acted as if under hypnosis.

With one hand she unbuttoned Mathew's shirt, then pulled down his trousers. Mathew was now so hard and so big that she simply could not resist but climbed on top of him.

Claire never thought that she would be so attracted to anybody like she felt at that moment.

Mathew, lying on his back, felt as if he was flying high up in the air and the engine of the flying machine was making huge noises and vibrated vigorously and he thought that he had died and was in heaven.

Claire had her first sexual experience quite a few years back but she never felt so elated as now.

'This is it! She kept hissing. 'This is it!'

She was grinding down on Mathew's pelvis as it

vibrated and with her hands she was grinding his chest, shoulders, stomach.

It was as though she wanted to eat his lips and swallow his tongue. His face was wet from her saliva and he continued to shake, at times so hard that Claire felt she was traveling so fast that the journey would never end. Finally after a short spell of increased shaking she felt getting very wet inside and Mathew's shaking easing and finally stopping. Her muscles slackened and she just lay on top of him.

Mathew was still large but soft by now and she moved her body gently left and right until the elation passed and then she lay down beside him.

For some time neither of them said anything and then Claire gave him a gentle kiss and said.

'Didn't expect we would do it on our first date Mathew but tell you what: I never experienced anything like this, I think it was perfect.'

'Same here,' said Mathew while in his head he wondered how such a sensation could exist.

He never had sex before although he red a lot and new the "facts of life", but no book said it would be like this.

'You go to the bathroom and I will heat up the takeaway.'

When Mathew came back from the bathroom, the

dinner was served and he sat down without uttering a single word. In fact he was so confused, his mind in the turmoil that he ate, finishing his plate and taking a couple of glasses of wine, Claire gave him, without even noticing what he was doing.

'Thank you for celebrating my birthday with me, Mathew, I really enjoyed the afternoon.'

'Yes I did as well, thank you, but I think I better go now.'

'Maybe we could have dinner again sometime Mathew, what do you say?'

'I think it would be nice.' Said Mathew and got up.

Mathew took his coat and Claire helped him put it on.

'Your trousers are all wrinkled,' said Claire with a giggle and tried to straighten the top part and by doing so touched his groin.

'Mathew you are still large.'

Claire started to move her hand up and down Mathew's front and felt wet and warm inside again while Mathew just stood there with his mouth slightly open.

Claire kept her hand gliding up and down his neck and gave him a gentle kiss on the mouth.

Mathew was by now large and hard again and Claire proceeded to take off his clothes one by one, this time without hurrying. When she finished undressing Mathew,

Claire undressed herself, took Mathew's hand and walked him to her bed.

This time she sat on Mathew, put him into her, took his hands and brought them to her breasts. When his hands touched her soft skin and the swollen nipples, he was back in his flying machine, shaking, and he didn't know whether he was all inside Claire or just part of him.. This time it lasted much longer and by the time she felt Mathew's shaking eased, she reached her highest climax ever.

Exhausted, she lay motionless on top of Mathew and whispered:

'I love you Mathew!'

It was not planned. She really felt it was love albeit physical if it could be described as such.

'Mathew, are you awake?'

'Of course I am!'

'I was in seventh heaven you know.'

But Mathew was baffled and tried to sort things out in his mind.

'This sexual activity is wonderful. Of course it is. But why did she say she loved me?' Only his parents used to say that and he never believe them either.

He wanted to ask her why did she say that but when he turned to look at her to ask her she was asleep.

Mathew was ready to get up and go home but felt

a bit lazy and decided to lie there for another couple of minutes.

When he woke up it was morning and, he could smell egg and bacon frying in the kitchen part of Claire's place.

'Morning my lover. Breakfast is ready and I hope you had a pleasant dream. Just to tell you that nobody slept in this bed with me until now.'

Mathew was only sixteen and Claire was like a big giant compared to him, but he liked being squashed, sucked and manhandled by her muscles making his stringy tendons into a soft dough.

In these moments his mind and his body separated and while the body was enjoying, the mind was in a state of detachment where it could create its own pleasures.

'Mrs Martin?'

'Yes!'

'Chief inspector Bryant, Shropshire Police and this is my assistant Mr Northcote. Is your husband at home please?'

'What is it Maura?'

'That's him, upstairs, just getting ready to go to work.'

'It is the Police, Geoff, they want to talk to you.'

'Bring them in then, I'll be down in a sec.'

'Come in please. What is it all about?'

'We'll wait till your husband comes down if that is all right?'

'Would you like a cup of tea or coffee?'

'No thanks, we won't stay long.'

'Mr Martin?'

'That's me,' said Geoff entering the sitting room. What can I do for you?'

'I understand you are the owner of the Round Hall and Mr Williams runs a show called "The Family show" there once a week.'

'I'll answer with two yes's. I am the owner and Mathew Williams performs at his own show as you said, chief inspector. Is there anything wrong?'

'Well, we received a report that Mr Williams's claim that he has an extraordinary memory is a fraud and that he is cheating the audience. Could you tell us anything about the young man?'

'Of course I can. He is a young man of, as you said, extraordinary memory, and I am sure of it because I tested him myself and I can vouch for him.'

'Mr Martin, because of the report of a fraud, we are obliged to investigate. Could you tell us when is Mr Williams performing again please?'

'The show runs once a week, on Saturdays. If you

want to speak to Mathew, he is meeting me at my office this morning.'

'Thank you Mr Martin. We will meet you there in, say, about an hour. I'm sorry to have disturbed your morning.'

'You see, after all, your young Mathew is not what he seems to be,' said his wife Maura after the policemen left.

'I'm sure he is genuine Maura and this will give him even more publicity especially when the name of the claimant is revealed.'

When Mathew arrived to Geoff Martin's office, in the Round Hall, the police were already there.

'Good morning Mathew, these are the police inspectors Mr Bryant and Mr Northcote. They would like to talk to you.'

'I am Mathew Williams. How can I help you?'

Mathew sat down and switched his mobile phone off.

'As we mentioned to Mr Martin, we received a complaint that your show is a fraud and that you are cheating by claiming that you have an extraordinary memory. You understand that we have to investigate such a complaint.'

'Of course. But how can you do that?'

'We cannot do any tests ourselves to prove one way or

the other. We have contacted the University of Wrexham and they have accepted our invitation to do the test at your next show.

If you have no objections, they would not interfere with the show, but would oversee the way you collect the data and use the same data throughout your show.'

'In fact I will enjoy the challenge', replied Mathew, 'but I would like to ask you something. After I prove my claim that the special memory I have is true, will I be told the name of the person that made the accusation?'

'I am afraid you will have to sort that out with a layer. On us is only to investigate the complaint as such.'

'I understand.'

'We'll see you on Saturday then. The people from the University of Wrexham appointed to do the overseeing will be introduced to you sometime before the start of your show. Thank you for your time Mr Williams, and thank you Mr Martin for letting us use your office.'

'Who do you think is trying to damage you, Mathew. Have you any idea?'

'None at all Mr Martin. So far I have not harmed a single sole.'

'Well, I know you are genuine, and I am looking forward to next Saturday. Now back to business I have made more money having a show once a week with you than when I used to be opened five days a week with the professional actors but, what is more important to me, I have enjoyed seeing so many families coming back to the Round Hall.'

'I'm glad we get on well. I have very few friends and I am sure you are one of the best. See you next Saturday Mr Martin.'

Mathew decided to walk back to the small flat he had rented after his parents agreed to let him live on his own. He brought with him his computer and there were times when he stayed in the flat for days.

Walking home he wandered who could be accusing him of cheating.

It must be somebody he doesn't know but probably met through the show, maybe somebody feeling bad about loosing money in the show?

'I have put a limit that could be placed on the outcome of my answer to £50 and so far nobody raised any questions. I think it will be fun to find out.'

When Mathew arrived to his flat, there was a note in his letterbox. It was from Claire asking him to give her a call.

He could not settle down to do any work and decided to call Claire.

'No wonder she came and left me a note. I switched off my mobile when I went to Mr Martin's office and forgot all about it later.'

'Mathew, thanks for the call. I need to talk to you, it is important. Can we meet tonight?'

'Yes of course. I am not doing anything today. Claire, is there anything wrong?'

'I don't know. You will have to tell me.'

'OK, I'll be here.'

'Shall I get a takeaway and bring it to your place, say at about five?'

'Yes, that will be fine. See you then.'

Mathew still wondered whether Claire's worries were connected to the visit by the police when she came in with the food.'

'Mathew', said Claire, putting her arms around his shoulders: 'I have done something wrong. I have hurt you without you knowing and I am very sorry.'

'Claire, I haven't eaten anything all day and I'm starving. Let us have the dinner first and then you tell me what happened.'

Mathew noticed tears in Claire's eyes and was sure that it was something to do with her job. She worked for a computer company where her brother Allen worked as well.

'Mathew I am sorry I hurt you, I really am.'

'Could you tell me what is the problem Claire, please?'

'Allen Randall is not my brother, he used to be my boyfriend before I met you'

Mathew went back in his thoughts to the first visit by Allen, Beth and Claire to his show and he still did not understand.

'But as you said, it was before we met.'

'Yes but I met you because of him.'

'Go on.'

'He wanted me to find out how do you manage to answer all the questions at your show. That is why I came to see you in the first place. But you and I got friendly and I fell for you. He has some kind of list of fifteen thousand words or something like that and said he put that together for his girlfriend's uncle Mr Martin who was supposed to have tested your memory.

And today he came to my office and told me that police will come to close the show. I am very sorry Mathew.'

When Mathew heard the word police, everything became clear and he started thinking about the show and how to react to Allen's accusations.

'I'm so sorry Mathew', her eyes full of tears, do you want me to leave now?'

'No, Claire, no. I'm glad you told me about Allen. If you are not his girl now that is all right with me.'

'But it will be my fault when your show closes.'

'Don't worry Claire the show will not close. This Allen is a very stupid man.'

'Mathew if you want us to part I will understand because I wasn't honest with you when we met.'

'Claire you did not hurt me. On the contrary you have been honest with me and I like that. I am not very good with words but can I say that we are better together than apart. I can relax only when I am with you and I feel that you like my company as well. Next Saturday the Show will, probably, attract more families than before and I will have to be fresh to memorise the extra data, but it is only Monday today and we can enjoy ourselves tonight. Let us go to your place and taste that strong drink that you gave me on your birthday.'

'My name is Mathew Williams. May I see Chief inspector Bryant please?'

'Could you tell me what is it about please?'

'It is in connection with next Saturday's performance at the Round Hall.'

'Will you take a seat please. I'll see if he is in?'

'Hello Mathew, have you come to confess? I hope not because when I met you my impression was that you were an honest lad.'

'No Mr Bryant, I came to ask you for a favour.'

'Could you tell me what it is?'

'Could you ask the people from the Wrexham University to use the official police paper that you can supply, so that the paper slips could be identified in case there is a query?'

'We have already done that and they have accepted. Is there anything else Mathew?'

'No, that is all Mr Bryant. Thank you very much. Actually there is something else. Is it possible not to mention the use of the official paper until the tests are completed?'

'That has been agreed as well Mathew. See you next Saturday.'

Mathew did not know what Allen could do but the idea of discrediting Allen appealed to him. First Allen tried to use Claire to his advantage and when failed, he is now trying to hurt Mathew.

'I am really looking forward to next Saturday's show and I hope people will enjoy it too.'

'Today is a special occasion for me', announced Mathew at the Family Show in the Round Hall.

'This is my twentieth show and I have a premonition that something nice will happen to me. But let me not delay the packed program. We have a special group of people from Wrexham for the first time and some of you have been here before.

May I take this opportunity to name three people

that changed my life: First, my friend David who encouraged me to use my memorizing ability and who helped me when I most needed help. Thank you David.

And Mathew pointed in the direction where David was sitting. Second, Mr Martin for trusting me and helping me establish this show. And finally, for me the most precious, my girlfriend Claire for coming into my life.

To start with the show, may I congratulate Mrs Herbert on her reaching three quarters of a century today. That is the nice lady in seat number 28F East Stand. Happy birthday Mrs Herbert.

And there are two more ladies celebrating their birthday today but I will only reveal their ages if they ask me to.

'I was told a few minutes ago that today's attendance is 1473 paying visitors which again is the record so far but it makes my task of remembering all the data so much harder.

This has been my longest speech ever so let us start with the questions please.'

'I have a question', came a shout. How many people here are called Mathew?'

'Not counting me and all those who have not paid for the entry, only two.'

'And how do we know that your answer is correct?'

'Because I said so!'

There was a loud laugh but the voice came back:

'But why do we have to believe you?'

'Because I remembered the names of all the people coming and only two said their names were Mathew, and they are, by coincidence three and four rows behind you.'

'Of course, if you don't believe me, let me ask all those called Mathew to stand up.'

The audience laughed and applauded and the ice was broken. There were many questions and some of the people went up to £40 thinking it might be possible this young boy could slip up and they could make a few pounds. But Mathew gave satisfactory answers to all the Questions.

'Mathew, my name is Robin Reid. Could you tell me how old is my youngest daughter? I am prepared to contribute £100 if you give the correct answer.'

Mathew opened his mouth to answer and then realized that it was a trick question. He looked at the speaker and said:

'I am afraid I can not Mr Reid,' and here Mathew paused on purpose for a second or two and continued:

'But I can say that your youngest daughter presently here in the Hall is, or better will be, sixteen on the seventeenth of next month.'

The audience went quiet and then Robin Reid said:

'You are right Mathew the £100 is yours.'

As the show progressed, Mathew felt that something should happen pretty soon and he was right. About quarter of an hour before the show was to end, Allen Randall called:

'Mathew, my name is Allen Randall, could you tell me what is my profession?'

'Well Mr Randall, today you are a teacher. At least that is what you stated on your entry slip.'

'That is not correct. I am a computer programmer and have been for the last six years. I think your memory is not as good as you claim, or is there something you have not told us?'

'No Mr Randall, today you are a teacher, or should I say you stated when you came that you were a teacher.'

'That is not true and I can prove it with my slip,' and Allen stood up holding the entry slip in his hand.

On the other side of the hall Claire started shaking. Oh God? Save my Mathew please?'

'Mr Randall,' said Mathew, 'you probably new that the police were contacted last week with a claim that my show is a fraud.

The police are actually here and with them are the scientists from the University of Wrexham. They can check your paper slip and confirm that either you or I are not telling the truth.'

'I am not afraid,' replied Allen and walked down to the stage, where the referees were sitting, and handed his paper slip.

'No Mr Randall,' said the spokesman for the panel after examining the slip. 'This is an ordinary paper. Today we have supplied special paper used by the police.

We can definitely say that you Mr Randall are the fraud and I am afraid to tell you that Mr Williams has our support if he decides to sue you.'

Allen Randall's face suddenly looked whiter that that of Mathew. He gave Mathew a quick glance, looked back at the panel and stormed out of the Round Hall.

'Ladies and Gentlemen,' started professor Horowitz, University of Wrexham have been invited by the local police to examine the claim by Mr Randall whom you saw leaving just now. The University appointed my colleagues here and me, from the Information Technology Department, and may I say that we are satisfied to the authenticity of Mr Williams's ability.

Thank you for your patience and cooperation and I hope you enjoyed the show as much as we did.'

While the audience was still on their way out, professor Horowitz approached Mathew:

'Mr Williams, or may I call you Mathew, I don't know what kind of brain you have but would you be interested in participating in research our department is currently involved in.

Due to the uniqueness of your ability you would, I believe, be offered a grant for a fixed duration, which could be quite substantial.'

'It is very flattering. I'd be thankful if you could prepare a proposal in as much detail as possible before I decide whether to participate or not.'

'I have to contact the Science Research Council so it might take two or three months and if everything is agreed, the research program could start in about six months from now.'

'I'm looking forward to your proposal professor Horowitz, and now will you excuse me please?'

'Yes of course Mathew.'

Mathew noticed Claire sitting alone in the stand and he waved for her to come down.

'Oh Mathew, I was very scared when Allen started accusing you. I thought something might go wrong.'

'It is all over now Claire. In a few days Allen will not pester you any more.'

'I am sorry Mathew.'

It was Geoff Martin, showing delight and anger at the same time. 'I never suspected Allen could do such a thing. I think our Beth is better off without him.'

'It doesn't matter Mr Martin. The audience loved it and I enjoyed it as well.'

And, for the first time, Mathew took Claire's hand and they walked out together.

'Claire, I am exhausted and need a good night's sleep. May I spend a night at your place?'

'You don't need to ask. My place is yours and I will make you something to eat before you fall asleep.'

'You know Claire, I was lucky to have met you.'

'Mathew, it is the nicest thing you ever said to me.' She squeezed his hand and they walked in silence the rest of the way.

In the morning there was the intercom and when Claire answered the voice asked:

'Miss Batersby?'

'Yes, who is it?'

'Foxley Motors. Is Mr Williams there please?'

'Hold on Claire, I will speak to them.'

'Hello, could you wait there please. I'll be down in a second.'

'What's it all about Mathew?'

'I won't be a minute. There is a parcel I ordered.'

After a few minutes when Mathew came back, Claire noticed he looked different. There was a change of colour as if he was blushing.

'You did not bring any parcel up Mathew. Could you tell me what was it all about?'

'Claire, tomorrow is your birthday but your present has arrived today. Happy birthday Claire!' And with that Mathew gave her an envelope in which there was a small key.

'Come to the window and have a look! This key will open the little thing parked down there.'

Claire was stunned. She looked at the key, then at the car and then at Mathew. Finally she put her arms around Mathew's shoulders and started to cry.

First it was a quiet sob and then it grew into an uncontrollable one, her arms gripping tightly around Mathew. It was such an experience for Mathew that he could not do anything but stand there not believing what he was witnessing.

After a while, Claire calmed down but kept her arms around Mathew.

'What was that all about?' whispered Mathew afraid that she might start again.

'Oh Mathew, and I thought you did not want me any more.' And after a pause she said: 'I am the happiest girl in the world.'

Since the departure of Steve, the house was actually very pleasant. When Tom did not want to learn new pieces, or practice the old ones, his mother would let him relax and she would sit and play for her own pleasure.

Not needing to concentrate to his mum's playing was the most pleasurable time for Tom. During these times he enjoyed music played to the full.

'Tom dear, I think this musical race is damaging your health. Maybe we better modify your performances so that you don't get so tired. And one other thing:

I started putting part of the money you get into a special account under your name and me as the guardian. This is so that your father could not demand part of what you earn.'

'Mum, why did dad leave without even saying anything to me? I didn't have an argument with him.'

'Tom, you are now sixteen and I think that you should be told the truth but first promise me you listen to the end before you react to what I tell you?'

'Of course mum, I have never been cross with you?'

'Tom, your dad and I could not have children for many years'

'I know that you were married for four years before I was born.'

'Yes Tom. Steve and I lived together for three years before we got married, so after seven years of me not being able to conceive, we decided to try and apply for the adoption.'

At this point Tom did not interrupt but waited for what was to come with fear in his heart. Irene paused for a few seconds and then putting her arm around Tom's shoulders continued:

'We put our names on the waiting list and soon there was a call, from the adoption agency, to go and see them. We were told that there was a baby available for adoption. As soon as we saw you we fell in love with you. The authorities told us that your mother, I mean birth mother, died at your birth.

So we adopted you and I became your real mother, and I still am and always will be.'

Here Irene gave Tom a tight squeeze and held him close to her.

Tom said nothing. He said nothing for some time and Irene noticed his face getting as pale as was the white shirt he was wearing. Then after a very long time he whispered:

'And what about my father?'

'We were told that your father died soon after your birth mother became pregnant. I'm sorry Tom. We should have told you this years ago but were always afraid the news could hurt you.'

'How is it then that I inherited your talent for music?'

'I don't know Tom but I am delighted you like the

music, especially classical music. It gives me strength and fills me with peace.'

'I am sorry that I can't read the music mum. If I could, you would have lots of free time.'

'We'll get on well together Tom, just the two of us', and they warmly embraced each other.

'Claire, you never mentioned your family. I keep going on about me and never even ask you about your parents and if you have any brothers or sisters.'

'The simplest answer is I don't know and I never will.'

'You must not say that. One day you may change your mind and….'

'Well, let me tell you what I do know! The first thing I remember from my childhood is a whole lot of children in the dormitory. That is where I started from, Mathew.

Then a family fostered me, but they had me only to get that extra money from the council. I was not treated badly there. Most of the time I, and there were two more girls, were left to amuse ourselves any way we knew.

Then when I was six, I was back in the children's home. I saw how some of the older girls worked at school and read and then left to a decent job, while others wasted their time and got nowhere so I decided to work. I have been on my own since I was sixteen and had a few boyfriends but always wanted to have my own place and I was never without a job. But I was always a loner, and when I met you I was just curious as to how you looked like I did when I was your age.

Then it happened!

After we spent our first night together at my place, you became part of me. One moment I was happy and saw myself waiting for you to come from work and we having dinner together and the next, I was afraid that it was only a one off for us.'

'But Claire you have not been adopted. Surely you didn't need to wait till you were eighteen to find out who your birth parents were.'

'No Mathew, when I was about two months old, I was left at the hospital entrance and my birth mother never came to claim me back. I was looked after by the hospital staff for a while before I was sent to a children's home.'

'I'm sorry. I didn't mean to bring it all up. Did it hurt you knowing that?'

'It did years ago, but I got used to it. I lived for myself and enjoyed learning shorthand and using word processor. After doing a number of jobs, I decided not to have a permanent job but do temping. I enjoyed my life and never thought I would fall in love.

Mathew I never thought I could feel for anybody as

I do for you. Do you know what I am saying? I love you and I always will. You make me happy and complete. It feels as if we are a real family.'

'But we are not married or anything like that, are we?'

I'm sorry Mathew I don't mean to tie you down.

'Claire, I'll be eighteen soon. You know I am resolute to find out about my mother, visit her grave and put a bunch of flowers on it. When I sort that out we can talk about our future but as it is now, you are everything I have.'

'And you are everything I ever wanted. It must have been our destiny to have met the way we did.'

'Claire, we are together every day and see each other more than many married people. Why don't we get a flat and live together. Looks like we both want that.'

'Mathew, my love, I was afraid to mention that in case you think I was over possessive. Yes, it would be lovely. We can go to the estate agent and see what is there available for renting.'

'But I was thinking that maybe we could pay a deposit and buy the flat jointly.'

'Come here my lover. If you only know how much I love you.'

And they joined in love as they did so often and with so much passion.

After looking for a place they could move in together, Claire and Mathew had an afternoon tea at a local coffee shop and went to Mathew's flat where he wanted to check further on flats availability on the internet. There was a letter in the mail box addressed to him with an official stamp.

Opening the letter he found that he had an appointment at the council offices with a councilor concerning his adoption and his birth parents.

'Come in Mathew. Please take a seat.

'My name is Carroll Paterson and I have been appointed as your counselor. I have invited you here because you have chosen to meet a counselor at the local authority.

I read all the correspondence you had with The General Register Office in Southport. May I ask you to show me an identification document such as your passport or a driving licence?'

'I brought my passport. I hope I don't need anything else.'

'No, passport is fine. Let me just take down the details and we can proceed with our meeting.'

'Well Mathew, when you supplied your details to The General Register Office, you stated that your mother died at your birth and you would like to know where she is buried.

I need to ask you if you are ready to take the information, I am going to give you, calmly and without the distress?'

'Of course I am ready. It all happened eighteen years ago.'

'Well, your original name was Mathew and your date of birth is as stated in your passport.'

'Now, your mother's name is Sharon and your father's name was Mike.'

Mathew twitched and froze. After a few seconds, he said.'

'Could you repeat that please. You said my mother's name is, and not, was Sharon?'

'Yes Mathew, up to last week when this document was sent to us here, your mother was still alive.'

'Are you all right Mathew. Can I bring you a glass of water?'

But Mathew did not hear. Since he found out that he was adopted, he believed his mother died when he, Mathew, was born and almost blamed himself for killing her.

Why did his adopted parents lie to him and told him his birth mother died at his birth?

'Mathew, I have called for an ambulance. Maybe it

would be better if we end the meeting for today and start again tomorrow if you agree.'

'No, we don't need to postpone this meeting. I had a shock hearing that my birth mother is still alive when I was told by my adopted parents that she died at my birth.'

'I am so sorry you were misinformed. Sometimes the notes get misplaced and the resulting confusion creates profound distress. I hope you soon find peace within yourself.'

'Has my mother ever tried to contact me? Why did she give me for adoption? Do I look like her or like my birth father? Questions like that are giving me a lot of pain.'

'Well, let me tell you what happens next:

If you want to proceed with the search, I can give you an application form and with it and the details I gave you, you can apply for a copy of your original birth record at any time you want. To try and contact your mother, there is a separate procedure.

For that, there are different ways you can take. One of them is the Adoption Contact Register, which puts adopted people and their birth parents or their relatives in touch with each other if this is what they both wish.

If you want, you can approach The Children Society. They would trace your mother and inform her that you would like to contact her. It is, then, up to her to agree and The Children Society would pass the information, she gives, to you.

This is called a step by step approach and, from my experience, the best way to proceed. Take these leaflets to read and here is the address of the Children Society.'

'I'll take your advice Mrs Paterson. Could you help me fill the form please and I'd be grateful if you can supply me with the Children Society address.'

'Of course Mathew; and if you need any help or advice in your search, I am always here for you.'

'This is brilliant mum. I wish we could live here forever. I feel so relaxed and have no aches.'

'Joe what are you talking about, what aches?'

'Oh nothing. Just that when I practice on the court I develop a headache and I could not think about anything else.

That is why I like it here. I don't need to think what I am doing.'

'When did you start having these headaches Joe?'

'I think about a year ago. First I thought I twisted my neck and it was stiff but the headache came back every time I started to hit the ball.'

'You should have told me about your pain. We will go and see the specialist as soon as we come home.'

'Yes mum, but let us enjoy all this. I'm going for a swim again. It is so nice just to sit in the shallow water and lift your legs and when the wave comes it simply turns you over as if you are doing head over heels backwards.'

'How Bert Langley saw Joe and assessed him down to the last detail', thought Ann.

'Joe looks clever, attractive and has a real sportsman's body. Yet he is like a child without any worries.

Maybe it would be good idea to take him for a check up. Up to now he had only physical tests. I think I will make an appointment with a psychologist. It might tell us something we do not know.

But let us have fun while we are here.'

Ann ran to where Joe was sitting, splashed him with water and started to swim without looking back.

'What have you done with Joe?'

Asked Paul the day after they came back. I have never seen him happier. He almost smiled at me first thing this morning.'

'Paul, these last two weeks made me realize that we don't really know Joe. He was as happy as a young child could be and yet I found out that he has a problem with his tennis. He told me that he gets headache whenever he plays or practices and I think we should take him to see a specialist.'

'But he has regular checkups with Bert or do you not trust that man?'

'No, not that sort of tests. I mean to take him to the psychologist, and maybe have a CT scan done as well.'

'What are you saying Ann? Joe is bursting with health, everybody can see that.'

'Yes, Paul, but only on the outside. We don't know what is happening inside his head, do we?'

'OK. You make an appointment with the specialist and for the scan but, I am sure, it is a waste of time.'

'I hope so Paul, I hope so.'

Ann decided to take Joe to a private clinic in Chester and have all the tests done in one place. She arranged everything by phone and she and Joe left early Monday morning and arrived at the clinic at ten o'clock.

The receptionist said everything was ready and they were introduced to the Consultant, Dr Nicholls.

'We, the traumatologist Dr Weatherill and myself thought it best to start with the physical examination but seeing Joe it almost looks a waste of time. Anyhow let us do that first.'

After the physical examination and muscle CT scan was complete Ann and Joe went to have lunch while the two specialists studied the results and compared their notes.

The afternoon was used to do a study of Joe's brain

impulses with Joe running on the thread mill at different speeds and slopes and finally the discussion with Joe about his life as a professional tennis player, its pleasures and agonies.

'Mrs Brown, we have done the analysis of the results and to tell you the truth we would like to recommend that you take Joe to London where he would have similar tests but with different instruments.

We have detected some changes in Joe's physic but it would need to be confirmed or disproved by alternative method to make sure the results are not giving us an incorrect picture.'

'Ann was listening and the longer the consultant's comments lasted the more confused she became.

'Could you tell me all that again but this time in a way that I can understand please?'

'Yes, of course, but you have to understand that we could not say that for sure. Joe looks one hundred per cent fit young man. The instruments, on the other hand show that his muscles are aging or should I say getting older.

We don't know why and how. The London clinic, we have in mind, has instruments that are somewhat different and when theirs and our results are compared, we believe that the diagnosis we have in mind can be confirmed. It would benefit if you could undergo the tests in London as soon as possible so that both tests are undertaken under similar conditions.'

'Dr Nicholls, I cannot follow your explanations but all I ask of you is: could you organize our visit to the clinic you have in mind and I can do the rest?'

'Yes of course, Mrs Brown. Give me ten minutes and I can give you all the details: Consultant's name, Clinic and the time of your appointment.'

'May I speak to Mrs Paterson please, my name is Mathew Williams.'

Mrs Paterson is out. Could she call you back Mr Williams?'

'Yes of course. She has my number. Any time will be fine with me.'

Mathew received his birth certificate and was all excited. It was true that he was born in South Birmingham Private Clinic as his adopted mother had told him, and the date of birth is the same as in his adoption documents.

His surname at birth was Osborne; his father's name was Mike. His parents were married, and lived in Bridgetown not too far from here. His mother was a secretary and his father a bank clerk. Before being married, his mother's surname was Leaver.

There were no previous children and his parents were married eight years before he Mathew was conceived.

'Mathew, this is Carol Paterson. What can I do for you?'

'Hello Mrs Paterson. Thank you for calling me back. I received my birth certificate and am very pleased. There is just one question. Why do they put the exact time of the day into the birth certificate? I thought the date would be sufficient?'

'Sometimes the time of birth is included as well. Could you come in and we can go through the details and see if there is anything else to be done? What about tomorrow morning?'

'I can make it tomorrow Mrs Paterson. Thank you.'

Mathew became suspicious.

'I told her everything was clear but she still wants to see me. 'I hope there are no obstacles, now when I came so far', thought Mathew.

'Mathew I am sorry you had to wait. I had a client that needed a lot of reassurance.'

'It's all right. I have lots of time.'

'Now, may I have a look at your birth certificate please?' As she looked at the document, Carol Paterson said to Mathew:

'You see Mathew, here it says no previous children, which is correct, but when the time of birth is entered it means, and I hope I am right here, that your mother might have had twins. Now Mathew do not take it as definite but I would like you to be prepared just in case that it is so.'

Poor Mathew could not move his eyes from the document. Up to ten days ago he was alone in the whole world and now he is supposed to have a mother and a brother, or is it a sister?

He did not see Carol leaving the interview room and coming back with a glass of water and a tablet in her hand.

'Here Mathew, take this and drink some water. I know it is a shock; that's why I wanted you to come here.'

'What do I do now Mrs Paterson?'

'What you should do does not change. You contact the Children Society and then you wait for their search. When they get anything, they will contact you. It usually takes up to a couple of weeks.'

'You are so good in calming me down. I am really grateful.'

'I know how you feel Mathew. I was adopted as well and had to wait till I was eighteen before I could do anything.'

'And were you ever sorry for trying to find out about your birth parents?'

'It was a mixed bag, so to say. My mother's parents contributed a lot for me to be given away but my father didn't want me either. But being brought up away from them makes me, in a way, different.

Your feelings, reactions, and your normal behaviour is different and very often adopted children don't get close to their birth families.

But every person is different and even you could not predict as to how you will react to whatever you find.'

'I am normally very calm but I started noticing lately that whenever I try to look into the future, I get a head-ache and could not think clearly.'

'Once you find all the facts about your family, you will be at peace with yourself and will feel much better, believe me.'

'I do Mrs Paterson. Thank you for everything.'

'Tom I am going to make an appointment to see our doctor, would you like me to make one for you as well?'

'Why mum, do you think I need to see him?'

'You seem to tire easily. Maybe the doctor can give you something to boost your energy. We are both work-ing and the late night shows take a lot out of both of us.'

'OK, if you think so mum.'

But Irene did not need to see the doctor for herself. She felt Tom looked run down although they have cut down the number of evenings Tom had to play.

When Irene played a new piece for Tom to learn, she noticed Tom needed a break after a relatively short time compared to what he used to.

'There is a change in Tom', thought Irene, 'instead of learning faster as he is older, sometimes he even needs to go through the musical piece more than once to be able to remember it properly.'

On the day of the doctor's appointment, Irene tried to explain the changes to her doctor.

As he was familiar with Tom's medical history, the doctor thought it better to refer him to a specialist, saying it could be a glandular fever but informing the consultant, where Tom was sent to, of the overall condition of the patient.

'I don't ache anywhere mum; I just get tired very quickly. Is that the symptom of glandular fever?'

'The doctor did mention that the new glandular fever virus causes no sore throat and that is why it is more difficult to diagnose.'

Irene did not want to worry Tom but she herself thought it better for Tom to do all the tests necessary.

Tom did not look forward to the trip to London.

He played there a few times and he and his mum took special bus from where they could see many places of interest but for Tom the whole journey was boring. He enjoyed a few visits to the opera though. There, he did not need to remember the music, and would feel fresh at the end.

'Young man, what we will do here is a few scans of your body, your head and then a few normal specialist examinations such as your brain activity and your muscle reaction to stimulants such as noise, light and fatigue.

It will last for just over two hours so if you don't need your mother, she may go and come back when you and me are finished with the tests?'

'Yes, mum, you go and look around the shops. You like that and it bores me.'

As Tom was, lying still, being moved through the Machine, he imagined his birth mother being in her coffin while he, Tom, was a little baby.

'Right young man, this part of the examination is done. Now the sister here will cover your head with this nice hat or you may say an army helmet, and then we will do the second part of the test.'

Tom was given different stimulants, for what he thought they were sugar, chocolate, salt, and some sort of drink, Tom thought, containing quinine.

'Do you ever do physical exercise Tom, you look as if you don't like any?'

'I don't. I feel stiff when I play the piano if I do.'

'Fair enough', said the consultant, 'but you might feel better in other ways if you do.'

'Well, that is about all Tom. You were very brave patient and I can see your mother has just arrived. We will analyse the CT scan data and your doctor in Lowestry will have the results within a week or so. Now can you wait outside and tell your mother to come in please?'

Irene could not be told much there and then except that Tom was physically somewhat underdeveloped and would need to start doing more of an effort to get stronger.

'I hope that from the tests we carried out, we can find out what we are looking for Mrs Taylor but from what I saw, Tom is not suffering from any illness that I can see.

But let us wait for the results of the tests.'

'How is it that one day you stand upright full of confidence and the next you feel you are carrying a bag of cement on your shoulders. There was always a distance in the relations between my adopted parents and me.

Then, after some years of frustration and wandering I met Claire and felt as if I found what I was missing, my family, somebody I am supposed to belong to. Now I am again in a limbo. My mother had been dead until I was eighteen and now she is alive.

I had no brother or sister and now I have although I don't know yet whether it is a brother or a sister, is he, or she, alive or dead. Will it be a new start for me or will I see only a mirage and not reality and whatever I see is not there but somewhere else.'

'Mathew dear, there is a letter for you from Mrs Paterson. I thought you sorted everything out the last time you met her?'

'I did indeed. Must be something she forgot to tell me.'

Mathew opened the letter without expecting much and yet he was puzzled with the content.

'I'd be grateful if you can give my secretary a call to arrange another meeting with me. Any morning except Friday would be fine with me.'

'She told me last time I was there, the Children Society would reply within a couple of weeks.

I thought it was up to me from now on but the only way to find out is to see her again.'

'Would you like me to go with you Mathew?'

'I don't want to trouble you Claire but, yes, I would like that very much.'

A whole week passed before Mathew and Claire could go together to see Carol Paterson and by then Mathew said to Claire he was "ready for anything".

'Mrs Paterson, this is Claire, my fiancée. Is it all right if she stays with me please?'

'Hello Claire! Of course she can stay Mathew, if you wish her to.'

'Mathew I wanted you to come here because the Children Society wrote to me and as I have been your counselor to start with I thought it might be better if I go with you through this part as well.'

'Do you mean to say there was a response. That they found where my mother is?'

'Well in a way yes, but there is a small problem.'

'She is still alive, isn't she?'

'Yes Mathew, she is although she has been in a hospital for a very long time.

Mathew squeezed Claire's hand really hard and said:

'Did they tell her about me?'

'Yes Mathew they did but not directly. Let me explain. The counselor asked if she had any children and her answer was that she had but they died at birth.'

Mathew could not hear any more words Carol Paterson uttered.

He interpreted the last sentence he heard in a way that his mother did not want to see him and the other child of hers.

When he opened his eyes, Mathew was lying in the first aid room with Claire beside him.

'Mathew dear, are you ill?'

But Mathew just stared ahead of him and mumbled:

'My mother doesn't want to know me!'

'No Mathew, you did not hear all Mrs Paterson said.

Your mother was told after you were born that the babies died. That was what she was told by the doctor from the clinic.'

Mathew's memory started recalling the events that occurred before he fainted. In a few minutes, he was back himself being able to analyze the information he received.

'So I do have a brother, or possibly a sister?'

'Mathew, are you sure you can continue, although it might be painful for you?'

'Yes Mrs Paterson, you can go ahead', said Mathew squeezing Claire's hand again.

'Well, let me start with your mother being pregnant and in hospital. She had not been well since your father died in a traffic accident, soon after the pregnancy was confirmed.

Your mother gave birth', and Carol looked at Mathew making sure he could take all this, to three little baby boys. You, Mathew, were born first followed by Tom and finally Joe. Your mother never saw the three of you as she was heavily sedated during and after the delivery.'

'Mrs Paterson, can you tell me if my two brothers are alive?'

'Yes Mathew, they are, but they had, like you, been adopted and all the adopted parents were told that your mother died when the three of you were born.'

Mathew stayed calm and in deep silence and after a while said:

'Why was my mother told the babies died? And why were the adopted parents lied to, as well?'

'I don't know that, Mathew, but that has to be cleared, I promise you.'

'And I have been accusing my adopted parents all this time of lying to me.'

'Mathew, your mother will need some time to recover from the shock of finding out that the three of you are alive.

Would you like me to carry on until the time comes for you to be able to meet her? Your brothers should have been contacted by now and I will have their response, I hope, soon.'

'Is my mother living alone or did she get married again?'

'No Mathew, your mother did not get married and she has been in hospital for most of the time since you were born.'

Mathew was, by now, quite strong and felt that it is not as dark as it looked just after he fainted.

'Yes, I would like very much if you can do all what is needed and let me know when you can involve me, and of course my Claire.'

Mathew had another set of bad news. His partner

and owner of The Round Hall, Geoff Martin phoned and said his wife Maura passed away peacefully in her sleep.

Mathew and Claire attended the funeral services and Mathew suggested canceling next Saturday's show but Geoff wouldn't have it.

'You know me Mathew: The show must go on. And Maura would have wanted it to go on as well'

It was exactly two weeks since Joe had his medical and now he and his mum were preparing to travel to London.

Joe was in London before when he played in a junior tournament at the Queen's Tennis Club but the schedule was so tight, Joe could not see any of the places he heard of when he was still in school.

This time his mother suggested they have a couple of extra days in London and take a few sightseeing tours.

At the age of eighteen, Joe had no girlfriend and only a few friends all connected to the game of tennis.

A number of girls tried to flirt with Joe but found him very immature.

He would not take a drink and liked being pampered with affection like when he was five or six years old.

It was nice not to play tennis for a few days and sitting beside his mum.

Joe enjoyed listening to his mother explaining

London's history as the bus traveled past famous places. As the bus stopped at The Albert Hall to pick up more tourists, a Japanese couple came upstairs and sat in front of Joe and Ann.

The woman must have been well over seven months pregnant and seeing her, Joe said to his mum:

'Was it hard for you carrying me in your tummy, mum?'

There and then, Ann decided it was time to tell Joe about his past. She was sure the time was right.

'Joe, let us get off here. I am hungry and there are some nice restaurants around here.'

Ann found a small place with plenty of empty tables.

'I'll have steak and chips and a glass of water please', said Joe to his mother, 'I feel a bit hungry.'

'Joe dear, let us talk about your past. I want to go back to the time when you were born', said Ann after the food was consumed.

'Is it because you saw that woman on the bus in front of us?'

'In a way yes Joe, but this may take some time so listen to me please!'

'Joe, your dad and I could not have children for a number of years. So two years before you were born we applied for adoption.'

'And then I was born. Was it a surprise mum?'

'Yes Joe it was but listen to me carefully please. We put our name on the adoption register and one day a call came for us to go to the clinic near Birmingham to meet a social worker to show us a baby available for adoption.

When we came there and looked at the baby, it was you Joe. We fell in love with you straight away and brought you home and you became our son.'

'But does it mean that I was not in your tummy at all?'

'That is right Joe. When you were born the woman, which had you in her tummy, died and you became our child, and still are. And we love you as much as if you came out of my tummy.'

'So that woman was my first mother. And what about her husband?'

'We were told that he died in a traffic accident soon after your first mother became pregnant.'

Joe became silent and started eating his fruit salad. But he could not swallow. And he did not eat his favorite, steak and chips. For the first time in his life Joe was forced to think. Or better, he could not disperse the thoughts coming into his head. He felt as if he had just lost his parents and felt very lonely. Then he saw Ann and the thoughts vanished and he said.

'So my first parents died and then I got you and dad as my second parents.

If I had any brothers or sisters, would you have taken them as well as me mum?'

'I don't know son. You were the only baby shown to us. Your dad and I tried to tell you all this many times as you were growing up but we always found an excuse to put it off.'

'I wonder if my first parents played tennis or whether I look like my first mother or my first father?'

Back in their hotel Joe was somewhat subdued and Ann asked him if he would like to go for a walk after dinner.

'No mum. I think I will have an early night. If we are finished at the clinic early enough, could we go home tomorrow please?'

'Of course Joe. I'll phone dad and he can meet us in Chester.

Telephoning Paul, Ann explained all about the adoption disclosure and how Joe took the news about his past or about his first parents as he called them so that when he picked them up at the Chester Railway station he was ready for anything.

But Joe did not bring the subject up for the whole journey and on arrival home went straight to bed saying he was very tired. In fact it was the very first time Joe felt weak and drained of energy he never lacked until now. And he was confused. What if his second parents die?

'What would happen then? He thought.

Ann went to the kitchen to make tea and sandwiches and Paul picked the mail from the floor and went to watch the news. Looking through the letters he called Ann:

'Ann, what are these letters about. One is addressed to us, one to Joe, and both are from The Children's Society?'

'Probably asking for donations as usual. Everybody is asking for money these days.'

But Paul had already opened the letter addressed to them and as he glanced through the text of the letter he did not notice his wife coming in with the sandwiches and tea.

'What is the matter Paul, you look as if you've seen a ghost?'

Paul gave the letter to Ann and went upstairs. He felt very confused.

'How was it possible for them to be told Joe's mother died giving birth and after so many years she is suddenly alive and well?'

Joe was his son and Paul was very proud of what Joe achieved. The Browns were such a happy family for the last eighteen years and now just one letter could spoil all the good times they have had. Then he remembered the letter for Joe and ran downstairs and there was Ann, her face white holding the letter in her hands.

'What shall we do Paul, what shall we do?'

'There is a letter for Joe. We have to give it to him Ann. We have to be honest with him. But maybe it would be better if we talk to him about the news first.'

'I can't Paul. I feel so weak.' And Ann started to cry believing everything around her was breaking up. Paul sat beside her trying to console her just as they heard Joe going to the bathroom.

Without a word they agreed to confront the situation now and Ann went upstairs and asked Joe if he could come down when he is finished in the bathroom.

'Joe darling', said Ann, 'come and sit here beside me.'

Joe wanted to go to sleep but he loved his parents and he obediently sat between them on the sofa.

'Joe remember we talked today about your first mother and how she died giving birth? Said Ann.

'Yes mum, I remember but it doesn't matter because I have you and dad and I don't want to change that because I love you both.'

'Joe your dad and I received some news today that may upset you. That's why we would like to talk to you first.

We received a letter from The Children's Society. This society tries to help make contact between the members of the family that were separated by adoption.'

'But why should that upset me? My first mum died and I have you and dad as my parents.'

'Yes Joe, this is what we were told when we took you as our son, but apparently there was a mistake and the letter we received today says your first mum is still alive.'

'But I don't want to change you. I want you to be my mum. I don't want any change.'

'Joe dear, there is a bit more to tell you. The letter says that you have two brothers as well. And they would like for the three of you to meet; but if you don't want, nobody can force you to do it. Do you understand that Joe?'

'Yes I understand ', said Joe and went to his bedroom without any further word.

Next morning Joe came downstairs and asked if he could see the letter and read it.

'Of course Joe but there is a letter for you as well, probably saying the same thing. Here, you read them both and we are here if you want to ask us anything.'

'I'll read them upstairs', said Joe and left the kitchen in a hurry.

After a period of about two hours, Ann was ready to go upstairs when she heard Joe's steps coming downstairs.

❋

'Oh. My God no, not another knock for my Tom.'

Irene had just opened a letter from the Children's Society addressed to Mr and Mrs Taylor and, as she read it, tears started running down her face.

'We have been instructed by Mathew Williams, the letter said, born Mathew Osborne, to try and trace Tom Osborne, the son of Sharon Osborne and one of the triplet brothers and we believe you are Tom's adopted parents.' Mrs Sharon Osborne gave birth to triplets in Hereditch private clinic:

Mathew, Tom and Joe.

The three boys were adopted respectively by different families. For reasons as yet not known to us, the mother was told the babies died at birth and the three adopting families were told the birth mother died giving birth without any reference to the triplets. It came to our attention the children's mother is alive and, the oldest child of the triplets called Mathew would like to meet his birth family.

Of course it is up to your son Tom to decide whether to accept the invitation for a meeting or to refuse, in which case Tom's and your addresses will not be revealed.'

Irene froze. For over eighteen years she loved Tom as

her son, being told he had no mother or any other family and now this.

'How will I tell Tom? What will it do to him? And yet I have to tell him, it is my duty to reveal all and be there for him when all this hits him. Poor Tom!'

At night Irene took the letter to bed and read it a number of times and every time it said the same:' Tom's birth mother is alive and he has two brothers.'

'Why would anybody give false information to Tom's birth mother and to the three families that adopted the three babies?'

Why would anybody be so cruel?

Irene waited for a couple of days and when she saw Tom rested and relaxed, she decided it was the right time to inform him.

'But why? Why is she alive now when she was dead for eighteen years? Where has she been all this time? And how is it I never heard I had two brothers?'

Tom read the letter for umpteenth time and then came to his mum and said:

'But I want you to be my mum. I don't want another; not now; not ever!'

'Tom dear, the best thing now is to leave it for a few days and then decide. You see it is up to you and only you, to decide what you want to do. Whatever you decide it will be all right with me.

I will support you all the way. I have been your mother and you my son for over eighteen years and nobody could deny us that. Tom and Irene embraced in silence and after a while Tom said:

'Mum whatever happens I know I love you and I am sure you love me too.'

It took Tom a whole week to go through the emotions that had affected him but at the end he said to Irene:

'I will go and meet my birth brothers and my birth mother.

I think that if I don't, I would always wonder and maybe feel guilty, but I would like you to go with me, at least to the first meeting. Will you mum?'

'Of course, Tom, dear. I'll do everything to make you happy.'

'Will you help me write a letter to the agency mum. I have never done anything like this before?'

While writing the letter, Irene and Tom shed tears in silence each one afraid that events in the near future might affect their relationship.

Irene was afraid Tom might find his birth family links stronger that his links with her and Tom was afraid Irene would be less close to him than she had been up to now.

After posting the letter, Tom hugged his mother and said:

'Mum, I don't want to appear at any concerts for a

while. Could we have a break from work and go some-where, as you say, to recharge our batteries please?'

'Of course Tom, but the concert in Birmingham, next Saturday, we must attend as the tickets have already been sold and if we cancel it, the organizers may sue us for breach of contract.'

Caroll Paterson was informed by the Children Society that Tom and Joe agreed to meet with Mathew although both expressed their wish to be accompanied by their adopted mothers. Caroll spent a couple of days trying to find a suitable place for the meeting and then suddenly an idea came to her head.

'Why not the place where the boys were born?'

She traveled to Hereditch and organized a private dining room in the Southern Hotel in Hereditch and made a provisional reservation for seven bedrooms for the night of the meeting.

She then prepared a very delicate letter explaining the detailed plan of the meeting from the arrival of the three parties, their accommodation, suggesting the topics of conversation, to the departure of the brothers and their adopted mothers.

As Caroll had done this quite a number of times in the past and had gone through the procedure as an adoptee herself, she felt confident in tackling the delicate points an adoptee must go through in such a meeting.

The place must be arranged so that no member of any group could feel inferior to anybody seated around the table and the bedrooms were to be spaced at relative distance from each other.

An early dinner was planned for the initial shock of facing the strangers/relatives to be minimized.

She, Caroll would talk if there appeared a pause and be invisible while the contacts existed within the group.

Yet among all the reunions Caroll had arranged in her job as a councilor, this one seemed the most delicate. All three brothers thought, up to a few weeks ago, they had no brothers and nor sisters.

There would have to be plans suggested of how and when they should meet their birth mother but that was a separate problem Caroll was able to solve.

As it was April, she suggested for the meeting to take place in June.

Hopefully the weather would be better then and the parties would, by then, get used to the idea that they had blood relatives and were going to meet them in person.

She checked the contents of the letters again addressed them to the three brothers knowing there were going to be many questions to be answered by the relevant authorities concerning the statements and false declarations of death of the birth mother and that of the three children.

Tom Taylor's letter confirmed his approval and acceptance of the place for the reunion and said his mother, Irene, would be coming with him.

Joe Brown's letter arrived last but he accepted the place of reunion saying it would be appropriate. His mother, Ann, was coming with him and staying during the reunion.

Caroll guessed that the letters were written by the mothers, and not the boys and she felt Tom's mother to be much warmer and closer to her son than Ann towards her son Joe but both were caring and loved their respective sons.

She then replied to the three brothers confirming the date and the place of the reunion and added suggesting the approximate timetable and her availability to all the participants.

Caroll had gone through so many meetings like the one planned but none had such clouds over the past as this one.

She thought to make the reunion somewhat easier by going to visit the boy's birth mother before the June date for the reunion.

There just might be an explanation as to why was the information regarding the deaths of the boys and subsequently the death of the birth mother given. It was very difficult to accept that an error occurred four times concerning one family, yet Caroll could not think of any other reason.

Dear Mrs Brown,

'We have received the results of your son's tests from the London Clinic and have done all the analysis and comparisons.

It would be good if you could make an appointment to come and see my colleague and myself at your convenience to discuss the results. Your son Joe doesn't need to come, as no further tests are required.'

The letter from the Chester Clinic did not give any other information concerning the two checkups Joe underwent, one in Chester and one in London.

'Paul, what do you think of this? It doesn't say that Joe is fine or that there is something wrong. I am going to call the clinic right away.'

'I told you it was a waste of time. Anybody can see Joe is a picture of health. They probably want to charge you for another consultation.'

But Ann's fears forced her to make the appointment. As the reunion day was approaching she decided to choose the date to go and see Mr Nicholls a week after the reunion to give Joe and herself time to recover.

Joe played in fewer tournaments for a while now and this made him somewhat happier. Ann noticed, washing his T-shirts and shorts, different, somewhat pungent, smell.

'Joe, are you taking a shower after your games. Your sweat is very smelly lately?'

'Of course I do, mum, and I use shower gel instead of the soap. I feel much more fresh that way.'

Ann started noticing changes, as well, in Joe's behaviour and she begun to write down the details hoping it might help the doctor diagnose whatever trouble Joe is experiencing.

She noticed Joe said he was tired for the first time when he was seventeen years old. Joe's body odour changed around his eighteenth birthday. He walks flat-footed first thing in the morning but that soon disappears.

There were quite a few small changes that only a mother could notice like Joe appearing getting lazy or doing things without any enthusiasm and so on.

Irene was aware of the pressure Tom was under and she reorganized the concert. Tom played alone only the compositions he felt at ease with and Irene took on herself to play the compositions Tom was not keen on. Although Tom was over eighteen now, with his pale face and small body, he was still an attraction for the audience and the shows always ended with an encore.

It was the beginning of May and Irene booked a fortnight's holiday for the two of them in Newquay, in Cornwall. She and Tom took a log cabin situated at the walking distance to the sea and consisting of two small bedrooms, kitchen and bathroom. The place could be heated by an electric fire only, and Tom enjoyed watching his mother putting pound coins into the electric meter.

It was Tom's duty to make sure they do not run out of pound coins. They ate most of their meals in the pub in the town and enjoyed a game of snooker in the pub's back room after their meal.

But most of the time they walked on the sand and when tired, they sat watching the surfers swimming out to sea and then surfing back on their boards. Neither of them mentioned the month of June and at the end of the two weeks there was actually a bit of colour on Tom's cheeks.

'Mum you know the blue dress you wore when we traveled to London last time?'

'Yes Tom, the one you told me I look lovely in. Why do you ask?'

'Could you wear it when we go to the reunion next month please?'

'Of course son and what would you like to wear?'

'My grey trousers and the navy blue jacket. It matches your dress and that makes me feel great.'

'I am so proud of you Tom.'

'And I am so proud of you mum.'

They were on their way back from Cornwall by coach and arrived home just in time to watch the new quiz from the local TV studio.

Tom was very keen not to miss it and Irene enjoyed watching her eighteen-year old son behaving as if he was ten years old. The quiz was simply a game where the TV host played a number of musical notes and the contestants had to repeat the notes on their instruments in sequence. If the right notes were produced, this led to the next step where a new set of musical notes increased by one were presented. The winner becomes the competitor reproducing the largest number of notes.

Tom would sit on the couch playing the notes on his harmonica and enjoying being the winner but scarred to even consider applying to participate in the contest.

As Tom run to the sitting room and switched the TV on, Irene collected the mail and went to the kitchen to make sandwiches.

While the kettle was boiling she looked at the mail and noticed there was a letter from Dr Hern.

She automatically opened the letter and read it. One sentence in the letter caught her eye straight away:

'All the test results were within normal for the age of your son except for his physic, which looks as being inherited.'

Irene stopped reading and took the two cups of tea and the sandwiches to the sitting room. After an hour of watching the quiz, Tom said good night and went to bed while Irene went to the kitchen to tidy up and finish reading the letters.

She was at ease now knowing that Tom was not ill and took Dr Hearn's letter to read it again. As she went on the letter continued:

'However, the NMR or as it is called now, CT scan, gave some concern which I would like to discuss with you when you next come to the surgery.'

'What sort of concern is he talking about? If the test results were normal, why should that give any concern?'

This was so much on her mind that before Tom got up the next morning she phoned the surgery and got an appointment with Dr Hearn for late afternoon.

After lunch Irene found an excuse saying she promised her friend Janet to go and visit her and left Tom to enjoy his free afternoon.

Coming to the surgery she only waited about ten minutes before Dr Hearn came out and invited her to his consultation room.

'I'm sorry if my letter appeared somewhat unclear but I thought it was better to talk to you here Mrs Brown.'

Doctor, could you explain to me please your concern regarding the CT scan my son Tom underwent.'

'Yes of course. Tom's tests all gave satisfactory results. These included blood, tissue, bones and internal organs.

However, the CT scan of the brain produced results that are not usually seen in Tom's age group. I know Tom has special talent for music and that was noticed in the images of the brain but there were a few small grey areas which only appear with people aged fifty or over.

These areas are known for the ability to remember. What the clinic in London suggests is to have another scan in twelve months time when a comparison can be made with the results obtained at your last visit there were two weeks ago. If the two scans are the same then there is no need to worry.'

'What if the scans differ; what would that mean?'

'Well I don't want to alarm you but if there is a difference, it would mean that Tom's brain is aging prematurely.'

Dr Hern waited for more questions but none came. Irene Brown was stunned by the statement.

She felt she was spinning around so fast that she could neither hear nor see anything around her. Dr Hern called his receptionist and asked to make a cup of tea for

Mrs Brown and waited for the shock to loosen the grip on his patient. After taking a few sips of tea, Irene was able to speak again.

'Is there any medicine or extra vitamins Tom should be taking for the next year?' asked Irene with fear in her voice.

'Vitamins are always worth taking but try make Tom develop an interest outside his music. Repetitive work is often affecting human brain activity. I will organize Tom's next appointment in London and will let you know. In the meantime let us not trouble Tom. He seems very happy and these are the best years of young man's life.'

When Irene came out of the surgery and found herself in the street, she didn't know what to do. There was a café across the road and she was almost hit by a car crossing the road.

A young waitress came to her table and waited but Irene did not response for some time before realizing where she was.

'Mathew, dear, come in please, come in!'

Amanda let Mathew in but as soon as she saw him her heart started beating faster than she ever experienced and her hands shook.

She was elated to see her son, Mathew, after he left the family house over two and half years ago but was afraid to show any emotion remembering how Mathew reacted to them.

'How are you Mathew? Your dad and, I mean Roger and I read a lot about your success with your show and were very proud of you.'

'I came to say I am very sorry to have accused you of lying to me about my birth mother.'

'It's all right Mathew, you weren't to know.'

'But I should have known. You were always honest with me and did everything for me as if I was your real son. I was the one behaving without any feelings. I must have inherited this from one of my birth parents.

The only excuse I have that I did not know any other way. I am very sorry.

Amanda felt silent. Mathew had changed. He never apologized for the sixteen years he was her son.

'Have you found out any more about your past, Mathew?'

'Yes, I found quite a lot. My birth mother is still alive but I haven't yet met her. And I have two brothers. I was born as one of the triplets and there is a reunion planned in June. After that I hope all the three of us will go and meet our birth mother who has been in hospital, I was told, for a long time.'

'I can't understand why then were we told your mother died?'

'Well, the councilor conducting the reunion programme, told me the other two adopted brothers' families were informed likewise and our birth mother was told the three of us died at birth and I want to find out the reason why all that happened.'

'Do you have any friends in Shrewsbury Mathew', asked Amanda trying to divert the conversation.

'Yes I have, but not many. I still like to be on my own when I work although I can mix a bit easier now. From next month, I hope to be working at the University of Wrexham as well.

They want to study my ability to memorise large amount of data, and will pay me well. There is something else I was going to tell you. I have a girlfriend.'

I know Mathew it was in our local paper. People here still remember you. You have really done well, what with your show and now the university. I am very proud of you Mathew. And I am glad you have a girlfriend.

'We are together for some time now and I am going to ask her to marry me.'

'I am very glad for you Mathew. I hope you'll be happy together.'

'If you and dad could forgive me for my behaviour, would you come to the wedding please?'

At this moment Amanda burst into a loud cry. She instinctively embraced Mathew and whispered:

'Oh Mathew, you'll always be my son. Always!

For a short second Mathew wanted to withdraw and excuse himself but managed to control his body and accepted his adopted mother's state as sincere.

Mathew could not let go and say the name mother or father so he asked:

'And how is everything then. Do you still get visitors from the University?'

'Not as much as when you were here Mathew. Your, I mean Roger has been a bit depressed and likes to be alone. But we do go for long walks every now and then.

Then an idea hit Amanda and she spoke without any thought:

'Mathew would you like to come for a meal one day, with your girlfriend? Her name is Claire isn't it?'

'Yes it is. I would like that very much but I would like to talk to her first if that is all right with you?'

'Of course it is. Please call me when you find a free Friday or Saturday evening.

It would be nice to have company again, especially you Mathew and your girlfriend, Claire.'

Amanda made Mathew a sandwich with peanut butter, his favourite, and the two of them chatted with Amanda careful not to touch any topic that might undo the thaw she noticed in Mathew's conversation with her. On the way out Mathew made an attempt to give Amanda a hug which made her cry again.

'My name is Caroll Paterson. I have been appointed as the councilor for the reunion of the Osborne family. Would it be possible to see Mrs Osborne please? Here are my papers to confirm my identity.'

The nurse looked at the papers with care and assuring herself of authenticity, said:

'Of course Mrs Paterson, Sharon Osborne is in the garden now. I'll ask a nurse to take you to her.'

'Mrs Osborne, here is Mrs Paterson, your councilor, to see you. Don't forget, the dinner is in half an hour.'

'I don't know about any councilor; why do I need one after all this time.'

'Mrs Osborne, do you recall a visit by one of my colleagues some three weeks ago asking about your triplets, born eighteen years ago?'

'Yes I do. I told her they died at birth but she said something like them being alive and wanting to come and see me and now I am not sure whether I dreamt all that or whether it really happened?'

'It must be heartbreaking for you after all these years Mrs Osborne but they are indeed alive. I don't know as to why you were told they died and I am determined to find out.

I am working for the local council in Shrewsbury, and am organizing a reunion of your three sons. After they meet, they would like, very much, to meet with you if that is your wish as well?'

Sharon Osborne went into a deep silence. She saw herself and her husband Mike and the three babies in the house in Bridgetown. She was cooking the dinner Mike was fixing the shed in the back garden while the three babies were sitting on the blanket in the middle of the freshly cut lawn. She saw the babies but not their faces.

Then she heard a voice calling her and she tried to answer the door but could not move. Slowly she came back and realized there was a lady sitting on her bed trying to say something to her. Sharon had her medicine about six hours ago and her brain was getting quite clear by now.

'You say my three babies are alive.' There was a long silence and then Sharon continued: 'They must be grown up boys by now. Let me see; yes they were born over eighteen years ago. But why was I told they died at birth? Why did they do that to me and to my boys?'

'Do you remember who told you about your babies being dead Mrs Osborne?'

'The doctors from the Clinic my husband and I were treated by for me to get pregnant of course.'

'Excuse me Mrs Paterson but Mrs Osborne is due for

her medicine and the lunch is ready', said nurse Ruth, the nurse in charge of the ward.

'If you would like to visit her again you may come on Friday morning or Monday afternoon.'

Caroll Paterson said goodbye to Sharon and on her way out she thanked the reception staff.

She felt as if something was not right being told by the nurse when to come for her next visit. But she discarded these thoughts as irrelevant. The mistake happened over eighteen years ago and now only the pain remains.

Claire was anxious about going to Mathew's adopted parents, especially after Mathew stayed away from them for such a long time, but she showed a brave face and suggested getting an appropriate present for the visit.

The day Mathew traveled to Wrexham University to discuss the possible contract, Claire went with him and spent her time searching for the ideas as to what kind of present to buy.

She almost gave up when the idea came to her head. Mathew mentioned once how his adopted mother talked about buying a new decanter for the drinks table and Claire found one in the shop. Mathew's adopted father was a mathematics teacher and Mathew mentioned a few days ago a new book on modern mathematics.

She went to Waterstones bookshop and they actually

had one in stock. Claire reserved it and said she and her partner would be back later. When Mathew finished at the University and they met, he was delighted and said how clever Claire was.

They went to get the book and the decanter and drove home to Shrewsbury.

They were to visit Roger and Amanda the following Saturday.

'Mathew dear there is one more thing you could do and I think it would be very appropriate.'

'I don't get it Claire!'

'You told me your two brothers are coming to the reunion with their adopted mothers?'

'Yes I did. So what?'

'Well, Mrs Williams would be touched and proud if you tell her you would very much like her to go with you.'

The apartment Mathew and Claire rented consisted of two large bedrooms, sitting room, dining room and a decent size kitchen. Claire was very proud to have a place of their own and in no time it was furnished and decorated. Mathew was really pleased the way Claire set the place up.

He used one of the bedrooms as his study and when a bookshelf was put up and stacked with his books,

Mathew saw himself looking at the bookshelf in his adopted father's study.

He saw his adopted mother coming up to say the dinner was ready and suddenly Mathew felt sorry for hurting her so often.

'Claire I see the reason to ask my adopted mother, so I'll ask her to go with us.'

'No Mathew, it wouldn't be fair on the others. You should go with your mother, just as the other two will. I'll be with you in my thoughts.'

'And what if she says no?'

'I don't believe she will say that, but if she does, you always have me.'

Mathew felt very awkward coming to the front door of the house he lived in for over fifteen years believing the people there were his parents. Holding his hand, Claire felt him shaking.

It was Amanda who came to the door.

'Hello Mathew, come in please. And this must be Claire.'

'Yes this is Claire, and Claire, this is my mum.'

'I'm pleased to meet you Mrs Williams', said Claire as she noticed tears in Amanda's eyes. But these were not sad tears. Amanda was shedding tears through the sudden delight. Mathew had just used the word mum. After over three and half years he is back, her Mathew, her son is back!

'Roger, Mathew is here.'

As Roger came to the hall Mathew noticed he aged quite a lot in the last three years.

His plentiful hair was all white and his face showed a lot of sadness. But physically, Roger was still tall and healthy although there was no vigour in his step.

'Hello Mathew, hello Claire, I heard a lot about you.'

'Hello Mr Williams, Mathew talked a lot about you as well.'

Everybody sat down in the sitting room and before anything was said, Amanda got up saying she had to check the oven.

'I'll see mum for a second' said Mathew and followed Amanda. In the kitchen, he said:

'Mum, I did not ask Claire to marry me yet. I want to go through the reunion first, but I need to ask you something: Would you go with me to the reunion. It is in Hereditch, in Southern Hotel and we would need to stay overnight?'

Mathew looked at Amanda's face. Her eyes filled with tears again. She hugged Mathew and whispered:

'Of course, my son, of course I will go with you.'

Amanda wiped off her tears, smiled and said: 'Now help me carry this tray to the sitting room.'

Claire and Roger had a nice uninterrupted chat for a few minutes, but they both noticed, when the tea was brought in, that Amanda's and Mathew's eyes were somewhat red.

'Roger, guess where Mathew and I are going?'

'No, but I know where you just came from', joked Roger.

'Mathew and I are going to the reunion where he will meet his two brothers. They will have their mothers with them as well.'

'I'm glad Mathew. I hope you will be able to find out everything that has been troubling you for such a long time.'

The conversation was very light and there was no tension in the air, not that Claire could notice. Then they gave the presents. Amanda replaced the decanter straight away and when Roger saw the book, he looked at Mathew and nodded with a smile.

When Amanda asked Mathew if he visited Claire's parents yet, Mathew looked at Claire and she proceeded to explain how she was left at the hospital entrance door and never found out about her mother or father.

This brought the conversation to a standstill. Claire

excused herself and went to the bathroom and Mathew quickly changed the subject:

'Dad, did mum tell you, I am going to be paid by the University of Wrexham. I will be going there two days a week and they'll do all sorts of tests on the memory part of my brain.'

'Yes, Amey told me. And Dr Horowitz mentioned it to me the other day. It's fantastic how you manage to keep all the details in your head.'

When Claire returned from the bathroom, Amanda asked her if she could help with coffee and the two of them had a chat in the kitchen.

The visit by Claire and Mathew was a huge success for all. Roger was delighted with the change he saw in Mathew but more than that he noticed a glow of happiness in Amanda's eyes. Claire was happy seeing Mathew happy and Mathew, well, he never felt more at ease than he did leaving the Williams house.

Irene and Tom took a taxi to Cheltenham and had lunch there while waiting for the coach from Bristol, via M5 motorway to Birmingham, which was to take them straight to Hereditch. There they took another taxi and reached the Southern Hotel at just after two pm.

Very few words were exchanged during the whole

journey but as soon as they checked in and went to their bedrooms, Tom came to his mother's bedroom.

'Mum, there was a letter for me. Maybe the reunion has been cancelled?'

'No Tom, it simply gives us sort of a timetable and there are badges so that all of us could recognize each other by just looking at the names.'

'Mum, I'm scarred.'

'Tom, there is nothing to be scarred of. It is still early so let us watch the TV for a while.'

There were cartoons, Tom's favourite pastime and he relaxed sitting on the couch holding his mother's hand.

'Now Tom, you go and have a shower, dress, and then come here at just after four. We will walk down and see what happens next.'

As they approached the hotel Bar, there was another woman with a young boy and seeing them, Irene felt her knees giving up strength. She took Tom's hand and steered him towards the couple.

'Hello, I'm Irene and this is Tom, my son.'

Amanda got up and looked at Tom in disbelief.

'Of course, hello, I'm Amanda and this is Mathew, my son. My God, they are identical, aren't they?'

Mathew was first to come out of the limbo and put forward his hand and said:

I'm Mathew, hello Tom!'

But Tom was stunned. He often sat in front of the mirror just before the start of piano playing concert and patiently waited for the make up lady to finish doing up his face and hair. Standing in front of Mathew was like looking at himself in the mirror.

'Hello Mathew!' whispered Tom and accepted the hand Mathew offered.

'I see you have already met. I am Caroll Paterson your councilor and sort of a guide at tonight's meeting. Mrs Brown and her son Joe have phoned saying they might be about ten minutes late due to an accident on the M54 motorway. May I order tea or coffee or even something stronger, we are all of age now?'

Everybody wanted tea and Caroll left but came back almost instantly.

'These are Ann and her son Joe, and these are Irene with her son Tom and Amanda with her son Mathew.'

Joe looked nothing like Mathew and Tom. He was blond while Tom and Mathew had dark hair. Joe was over six feet tall and weighted almost as much as Tom and Mathew together.

'I play tennis.' Said Joe when everybody sat down.

'Tom is a piano player' added Irene hoping that the conversation would continue.

'Mathew has his own show on the stage and will soon start at the University' said Amanda.

'Mums, what about the four of us going to the bar and have a drink and leave the three brothers to find their own subject of conversation?' suggested Irene.

'They will be fine', said Caroll, 'We are the ones that need a drink to give us courage to help if we are required to, so let us give them some time alone please.'

Hearing the word brothers made the three boys speechless for almost a whole minute.

It was Joe who broke the ice saying:

'I started to play tennis when I was only five but now I don't like it as much as I used to.'

'My mother was a music teacher and I started to play the piano when I was very small. I used to like to perform on the stage, but lately I am getting tired learning new pieces.'

Mathew listened and absorbed the conversation but only said:

'I earn my money by being able to memorize everything I read or see.

None of them mentioned the word brothers. It was like thinking aloud without noticing anybody being present and listening, when finally Caroll came and said the dinner was about to be served and asked the boys to join her and their mothers.

Caroll very cleverly organized a round table with seven seats. She marked the seats with names in sequence:

Joe, Ann, Irene, Tom, Amanda, Mathew and herself, so that each of the boys sat beside his mother and none of his brother. This gave the boys a sense of security and yet they were facing each other around the table.

'Isn't it fascinating that none of the boys drink alcohol', said Ann to Irene, sitting beside her.

'Ladies and gentlemen', started Caroll raising her glass: 'welcome to your first reunion.

I am here only as the coordinator and only for this reunion and when the three brothers meet their birth mother. At that point my work will terminate and it will be up to the individual members to decide their future.

May I continue to say that I have visited your birth mother in hospital where she has been hospitalized for fifteen out of the last eighteen years. She is under constant medication but I noticed that just before taking medicine, her reasoning ability is almost normal.

She was very confused hearing about the sons she has but she is ready to see the three of you. Of course it is up to each of you to decide what to do. When I get the answers from all of you I will proceed to organize the meeting which, I am sure you'll understand, will take place in her hospital. And now let us enjoy our dinner.'

By having one adopted child and no children of their own, the mothers had something in common and they soon established a few topics of conversation. Boys, on the other hand, took much longer to start their small talk.

After dinner the mothers went to the bar and enjoyed a drink with a gossip, mostly talking about their sons' childhood.

For the three boys it was like looking out through the shut window. Safe beside their mothers yet close enough to everybody to be able to hear and see everything and everybody. Most of the conversation was between the mothers. Caroll sat contented and kept observing the boys and their mothers and thinking.

'Sometimes the faith could be very cruel, and it definitely was for this lot.

Amanda was very gentle and her face showed happiness although there were lines on her face expressing the sorrow of the recent past.

Irene showed concern about her son but was cheerful and enjoyed the evening.

Ann did not project much. There were moments during the evening when she looked like a professional agent or manager but she did keep an eye on Joe all the time.

The boys started, rather slowly, to exchange glances and there were occasional questions or comments and as the dinner was coming to an end, Caroll suggested a drink at the bar for the mums and the boys got up and moved to the TV room.

There were no other visitors there and the brothers relaxed and talked about their past and each praising his own adopted mother. But because they were always guided, except Mathew, there were no long discussions. There were no laughs or giggles heard from the TV room.

Mothers, on the other hand, were full of questions and comparisons were made all the time. They felt that, although their sons never new their brothers and had nothing in common, there were so many similarities.

'I notice that none of them laughs and they all like being alone', commented Irene.

'They seem to be very good but only in one thing. Isn't it curious', said Ann.

'Ladies, I think I'll call it a day and go to my room. Tomorrow morning at breakfast I would like to suggest a date for their, and our, meeting with the birth mother and then we conclude the reunion. I hope the boys will feel better for all this and if you or your sons need to ask me anything you have my address and my telephone number.'

'Thank you Mrs Paterson', said Irene. I think we should play it by ear and see how our sons react.'

'May I say that the hospital your mother is in is only about twenty minutes drive from here, but I'll give you all the details in writing.'

The morning was very much like the dinner. No

closer contacts were made and after Caroll suggested the date for the meeting with the boys' birth mother and it was accepted, the party ended with polite goodbyes.

Caroll did not want to prolong the waiting so the second reunion, the meeting with the birth mother, was set for the last week of June. She went to visit Mrs Osborne again just to make sure she will be well for the meeting. To her surprise Sharon was bright and looking forward to meeting her sons she had never seen before.

When the day finally arrived, the boys with their mothers, met at the hospital car park. Caroll took the brothers to the reception desk and a nurse took them to the meeting room. Caroll went to Sharon's room and found her ready and waiting but shaking with anxiety.

She walked with her to the meeting room and introduced her to the boys. There were no reactions from her sons except that they got up from their seats. Caroll held Sharon's hand and said:

'Mrs Osborne, these are Joe, Mathew and Tom, and boys, this is Sharon, Your birth mother.'

There was silence and Caroll, expecting this, continued:

'What I suggest is for Sharon to sit with you and tell you her story. It may give you some idea of the reasons why all this happened to you as a family. I will take your other mothers to lunch and we'll give you about two hours.

The nurse will bring some food so you don't need to leave until we come back.

The mothers were invited by Caroll to join her for lunch, which they accepted, and the boys were left, to face the meeting with their birth mother, alone.

Sharon's voice trembled as she started talking to her sons she saw for the first time.

'Mike, your father, was a very nice man. He was a large man with thick black curly hair, which he kept combed back. And he had a special voice, deep voice, almost hypnotic and listening to it was like listening to a Frenchman whispering intimate thoughts to his lover.

We tried to have children for a number of years and each of us felt guilty for me not getting pregnant.

About four years before you were born your dad developed severe heart problems. First he had sore throat, which would not get any better. Then after many visits to the doctor and the hospital the doctors told us that it was not a cold but rheumatic fever but by then his heart was diseased, the doctors called it the pericardial effusion.

They told us that with proper medicine he could even outlive me, so we decided to see if the IVF was possible.

For a few years previously I tried all sorts of medicines to see if I could get pregnant but at the end we made an appointment to visit a clinic. When we were told how much it would cost I cried and your dad was taken to hospital and they kept him in for three days until his heart settled.

We must have visited half a dozen clinics and they all quoted similar costs, which your dad and I could not afford so that was it.

A few weeks later we had a call from the director of a clinic, nor less. He asked if he could come and talk to us to which we agreed not knowing what it was about.

When he came, there was another doctor with him, sounded like American. They told us that there is a project sponsored by a very big medical firm and that not only we would not need to pay for the fertilization but the company would give us a one off payment. When they mentioned the figure we were to get and not paying anything to have a baby, we agreed and signed all the papers that they brought with them.

'But why would they pay you when, normally, there was a charge to have the IVF treatment?, asked Mathew.

'Well, we didn't think much about that. We were over the moon that finally we might be able to have children of our own. I was to have a medical and some gynaeco-logical tests and take the medicine they'll prescribe prior to the IVF treatment.

Your dad and I thought, we would be able to bring

up our child with the money we got and we put it into the bank for that purpose.

I was, at that time, on different medicines to your father and was taking insulin for my diabetes as well as tranquillizers. We showed the doctors from the clinic our medicines and were told that they will supply us with new drugs that will replace all that we were taking up to then. For the next six weeks we had to visit the clinic every morning and take the medicines provided.

After the six weeks passed, the IVF treatment started and now we were to start taking varied medicine again every morning.

After another few weeks passed we were called to the doctor's office and were told that unofficially I was pregnant.

Then the tragedy struck. Your father was walking home from the hospital when a lorry lost control, mounted the pavement, and struck your dad.

He died the same day he heard he was going to be a father. Hearing about the tragedy I fell into a deep depression and was given yet more medicine.

When I was about twelve weeks pregnant and was examined I was told that something was not right and they recommended termination of the pregnancy.

I then called a friend, Carl Campbell who was a lawyer and a school friend of your father's and when he came to the clinic and threatened to sue them, they agreed to the continuation of my pregnancy and Carl arranged for me to go to a maternity hospital where I was examined and sent home.

The pregnancy almost killed me. I had to take more medicine and at the end I was hospitalised, being sedated for the duration of the pregnancy. When I recovered from my depression I was told that I had triplets and that they died at birth. That finally put me into this mental hospital where I have been for most of the last eighteen years, which must be your age now.

'Do you remember the name of the hospital we were born in?' asked Mathew.

'I am sorry boys but they have numbed my memory with all the drugs I was given. The name seems as if called American clinic or something like that but I am not sure of anything anymore.'

Do you remember the house you used to live in, I believe it was in Bridgetown?'

'Oh yes, Mike, your father and I spent many happy years there but everything is like in a haze. The only place you could find anything of use might be in my suitcase.'

Up to then Sharon was steady and quiet but when she finished her sad story, she started first to sob and then went into an uncontrollable cry that lasted for a long time. Tom was first to sit on the chair beside her and give her a hug followed by Joe.

Mathew just stood there and his brain traveled in top gear back and fro covering the troubled years of his mother and the entire life, so far, of the three brothers. There was no sadness or pity in his heart, only anger and hate. He new why he was angry but he wondered who were all those people he hated so much.

'Do you remember the location of the clinic or where it was?' Mathew managed to ask.

'I'm sorry boys. I think the drugs have destroyed my brain. But Carl should know if you would be able to find him. I have not seen him for a long time.'

'And the names of the doctors? Can you recall any of the names from the clinic?'

Mathew could not use the name mother. He could not see either Joe or Tom as his brothers and the people he new as his parents and who became complete strangers to him are now back as the only relations.

In fact the only person he could tolerate near him was Claire and the only male friend he has ever had was David.

David and Mathew were opened with each other and Claire takes him as he is, doesn't praise or criticize him and doesn't try to give him any advice.

'Did Carl Campbell have his own office or did he work for a company?'

'I think there was a name Campbell & Campbell or something like that, but I am not sure of anything any more.'

'Do you have any papers that I can look through? There might be something about the clinic or the doctors involved. I would like very much to look through any correspondence.'

'There was actually a letter from Carl Campbell to your father somewhere in my case, but it was a very long time ago.'

'I'm sorry boys but your mother needs a rest now. She gets tired easily and your visit has made her tired. But you can come again next week, same time, if you like', said the senior nurse.

Tom and Joe gave their mother a kiss and the three boys left the hospital.

Mathew did not trust the nurse that asked the three boys to leave and he decided to play her game. He saw a label on her coat saying her name was Ruth and three days later came back to the hospital reception desk and asked when is nurse Ruth on duty again.

'She is on night duty all this week', said the receptionist. 'If you want to see her, you'll have to wait till next week.'

'I'll do that, thank you very much', said Mathew and left.

He came in, the very next day, during visiting hours and sat beside his birth mother.

'Let us see if you need anything', and he opened the suitcase under the bed and took out all the paperwork that he could see.

'I think you need some envelopes, writing paper and a nice pen so that you can write to the people you remember. And maybe some fruit for you to nibble at. I'll bring everything when we all come again.'

Mathew could not breath properly until he came home and put all the material from his mother's suitcase on the table.

There were many copies of the letters she and Mike sent to different hospitals and clinics. Some of them had replies attached to them and as Mathew read through, he suddenly felt sorry for his birth parents. Every reply was either negative or the cost was so high that it terminated the correspondence.

Then there was a bank receipt for twenty thousand pounds deposited into their joint account. He grabbed it and read the name of the bank "The First New York Bank" it said, and Mathew was sure that he could now trace the Clinic that destroyed his parents. There was an unopened letter from Carl Campbell and Mathew decided to open it.

A short note only inside, informing her that he was finally moving to France but, if she ever needed a solicitor, to call his former office and they would look after her. Mathew realized that when this letter came, his mother was already in quite a bad state, and never new why Carl stopped calling on her.

There was a photo of his parents on the beach in Blackpool. He new it was them because it said on the back of the photo: "Sharon and Mike, second honeymoon". The rest of the paperwork did not seem important at the moment but Mathew nevertheless sorted it all and filed everything methodically and placed all the original papers in a separate envelope marked "Osborne documents."

Something else puzzled Mathew. He visited his birth mother twice and during the first visit, when the three of them came, she was quite slow in her answers as if the medication made her drowsy. During his second visit she was able to talk more precisely about her past. Is it because of the medication or because she can communicate only with one person at the time, Mathew wondered.

Good morning. I made an appointment to see a solicitor please. My name is Mathew Williams.

'Please take a seat Mr Williams. You'll see Mr Tompkins as soon as he is free.'

Mathew was aware that he had been observed because after the secretary informed Mr Tompkins of his arrival, the camera on the wall turned and pointed in his direction.

He made himself look calm when Mr Tompkins appeared and invited Mathew to his office and offered him a seat.

'As our secretary explained to you over the phone our introductory offer is up to half an hour free consultation and thereafter our normal charges apply. Now, how can we help?'

'Mr Tompkins, my mother died when I was born and I was fostered and later adopted.

My adopted parents gave me my mother's correspondence about a month ago when I was eighteen. In the letters my mother mentioned Mr Carl Campbell as her and my late father's solicitor. I believe that these offices used to be Campbell & Campbell. I would be grateful if you could help me find where Mr Carl Campbell is now. My father and Carl Campbell were very good friends and I would like to know what was my father like. He died before I was born.'

'These were indeed the offices of Campbell & Campbell and Carl Campbell was a senior partner here.

We bought the business some 13 years ago and as far as I know Carl Campbell went to live in France with his second wife.

His first wife and daughter died in a traffic accident a couple of years previously. We kept in touch for a few years and I might have one or two of his letters at home. I will look for them and if I find anything I'll be glad to send you the details of his address. Could you leave your address with the secretary on your way out.'

'Thank you very much Mr Tompkins, and may I ask if you would represent me if I ever need a solicitor?'

'I'll be glad to do so Mr Williams, and I hope I have been of assistance.'

Indeed, not a week passed and Mathew received a letter from Mr Tompkins enclosing Carl Campbell's address:

Mr Carl Campbell,

84 Rue de Pintamont,

St Denis-d'Oleron,

Ile d'Oleron,

France

Mathew wrote to Mr Tompkins and thanked him for the information. He said, in his reply, he would try and contact Carl Campbell to ask if it would be all right to arrange to go over and see him.

'Directory Enquiries, International Numbers!'

'Can you find a telephone number for an address in France for me, please.'

'What is the address please?'

Mathew was so tight that he was surprised when the operator's recorded voice came on, giving him the number and the local code for the address he supplied.

He wrote down the number and tried to relax before deciding to make the call.

But he could not relax. He needed to be at ease or at least to act as if he was. To contact his birth father's friend without warning might raise doubt in Carl's mind and Carl might not want to meet him and that would not help find answers Mathew was looking for so, Mathew decided to give himself another day before making that call to France.

The following morning Mathew was ready. He dialed and waited and when the reply came it was a female voice speaking French. But Mathew expected that and said in English:

'I am calling from England. May I speak to Mr Carl Campbell please?'

'One moment please!' said the female voice in perfect English and there was a long pause.

'Carl Campbell speaking, what can I do for you?'

'Oh Hello Mr Campbell. May I take a couple of minutes from your time please?'

'Yes, of course. What is it about?'

I understand you were a friend of late Mike Osborne and his wife Sharon. Mr Campbell, I am their son Mathew. I wonder if it would be possible to come over to France and talk to you about my father I never met?'

'Mike Osborne! Of course Mathew, my wife and I are both retired and have plenty of time. You tell me when you are coming and I'll make sure we are at home.'

'Thank you Mr Campbell, I'll write and let you know when I sort out my traveling arrangements.'

'Looking forward to seeing you Mathew.'

'Mathew, there is a large envelope for you, with The University of Wrexham label on it but don't read it now as the dinner is ready and it is your favourite."

After dinner Mathew studied the letter from Dr Horowitz and finding it acceptable said:

'Claire, I will have to travel to Wrexham University twice a week for the next three years.'

'So you are to become a student', said Claire with a trace of sadness in her voice.

'No I am not. They will pay me sixteen thousand pounds a year to be there two days a week. They want to study my brain to try and find out how I could remember so much.'

Mathew run the few steps towards Claire and said:

'Now we can definitely get our own place Claire. He kissed her lips with such passion it surprised them both.

'Three years contract, it says, which means that we can look for something really nice.

'Mathew you are brilliant. What else do you have up your sleeve?'

'Well I have something as a matter of fact. We are now together for over two years and I think we deserve a holiday.

'What will your work consists of at the University Mathew?'

'Professor Horowitz says they would give me things to remember by reading. While I read, the instruments will monitor my brain activity. Then after a period of time I will have to retrieve the information from my memory and the instruments will again monitor my brain activity.

The material I will have to remember will vary from plain text to pictures, symbols, words in foreign languages and equations.

These include visual memorizing. I might have to do memorizing of sound signals as well but it doesn't say here anything about that so I presume there might be another agreement after this one terminates.'

'I didn't understand much of what you told me but I can see you are delighted and I am proud of you. Now you tell me what would you like for your pudding?'

After dinner Claire was somewhat quiet so Mathew got up from his writing desk, gave her a kiss and said:

'Claire do you recall I went to see a solicitor to try and find out if they can trace my mother's solicitor.'

Yes, I remember. You said they will try to get his address for you.'

'And they did. He lives in France. Would you like to go with me, when I arrange a meeting with him, please.'

Claire looked at Mathew trying to say something, but Mathew interrupted:

'It could be our honeymoon and our first trip abroad.'

'Mathew, are you…?'

'Yes I am Claire. We are everything else but married, so let us be that as well. What do you say?'

'Yes Mathew, I would like that very much.'

And tears started running down Claire's face.

'Are you all right Claire', asked Mathew.

'Yes, I am Mathew', whispered Claire.

'First time we were together I called you "my lover"

but the last two years meant so much to me. I didn't know one could be as happy as I have been.'

'Mr Nicholls and Mr Weatherill will see you now Mrs Brown' said the receptionist soon after Ann came to the clinic.

Ann entered the surgery with the intention to show displeasure of being treated like a NHS patient while paying high fees but Mr Nichols's approach dissuaded her and she accepted the seat offered to her and sat down.

At the same time Mr Weatherill came in from the adjacent office greeting Ann with a smile.

'Mrs Brown, first let me apologize for the way I wrote the letter but it was really best that you came in person.'

'Could you tell me as to why I had to come and not being told in writing?'

Ann was showing her anger but it was anger driven by fear, fear of unknown.

'Yes of course, Mrs Brown. Let me get straight to the point. Joe looks and feels as healthy as any sportsman would like to feel. But the test in London showed something we and our colleagues in London are concerned about.'

'So there is something to worry about?'

'In a way, yes. Let Mr Weatherill explain to you'

Mrs Brown, as you probably know a small mass

of our body with a nucleus is called a cell. During the growth of a person the human cell production is larger than cell loss.

In adult life, when physical growth stops, the balance is established, by complex control mechanisms, which evenly balance the continuing formation of new cells with cell loss. In old age, cell loss outweighs cell formation.'

'I'm with you so far', said Ann.

'With Joe we, or better the instruments, noticed that his cell production still balances his cell loss. But the process differs very much comparing with an average human of the same age as your son. This indicates that his aging will appear sooner than it does in normal circumstances.'

'Is there a name for such a case or is it called a disease at all?'

'No there is no name and we don't know why it is happening.'

'So what is your conclusion, what is going to happen to Joe?'

'To be honest we do not know but we think that Joe will age much faster than an average man does. Physically, Joe's state would indicate, according to the instruments reading, without knowing him personally, to be about thirty five to forty years old. We would like, very much, to be wrong but the indications tell us otherwise.'

Ann sat in the chair, her mind racing through the last eighteen years of her life and the whole of Joe's. Why, why should this happen to Joe? He had been handicapped enough with low intellect and other mental qualities. His body is all he has and all he can use. It is not fair. Not fair at all.

'Would you like to ask us anything Mrs Brown', asked Mr Nicholls.

'How do we stop it', wanted to ask Ann but at the end she just whispered:

'I don't know what to do now. I love my Joe you know and I would do everything I could to help him.'

'Mrs Brown, all the data we collected on Joe are stored and what we suggest is that you keep a diary and record any changes you see in Joe.

Then after a year or so we would like him to have the same tests he underwent in London. After that we hope, we would be able to tell you more when we compare the results of the two tests.'

'Should Joe stop playing tennis and take it easy. Would that help?'

'If we know the cause of this happening, we would have the answer. But as it is, with all honesty, we really don't know.'

Ann had to stop a number of times driving back to Cranspole. She saw, in her mind, Joe and Paul sitting in front of TV and Joe looking older than his father.

On her arrival, Joe and Paul played table football using pound coins as players and small shirt button as a ball.

Seeing Joe so happy, Ann's fears suddenly disappeared and she was sure that next year's tests results would prove the doctors wrong.

'Well, have you found out anything new with your specialists, as you call them?'

'No Paul', answered Ann 'not much.'

'I have an appointment to see professor Richardson please, my name is Williams, Mathew Williams.'

Oh, yes Mr Williams', said the secretary. 'Could you take a seat please, professor Richardson will see you as soon as he is free.'

Mathew has read a lot about the IVF and could not see any connection between it and the disproportions of the abilities in himself and his two brothers. He hoped this visit might give him at least a lead and guide him in his search for the answers he craved for.

Professor Richardson was one of the "old guard" medical scientists very much against the research in creating designer babies. When he received Mathew's letter, his mind went back in time to the second half of the last century and the trend in medical research undertaken by the leading pharmaceutical laboratories.

Many scientists were lured to come and work in these laboratories by the most modern equipment and huge salaries.

He was one of the few to have refused the invitation. Scientists who worked there were not allowed to submit any results for publication unless their employers approved first, so very little was published and very little was known about the work in these laboratories.

There were rumours that many pregnancies had spon-taneous abortions and many were terminated in order to study the effects of the chemicals on the foetus's physical development. But no results, in that field were ever published.

'This young man, Mathew, must be one of those that were born about then and I would like to find out more about what happened', thought professor Richardson, when his secretary came in and said that Mathew Williams is in the waiting room.

'Bring him in Alice please, I'll see him now.'

Alice Freeman was professor Richardson's secretary for the last seven years and during all that time she never witnessed a young man coming to the surgery. Consultant gynecologist sees couples or single females;

very seldom single men and, she never witnessed a visit by a man of such a young age. Yet she thought that this young man looked very familiar, as if she had seen him before. Professor Richardson showed a very keen interest in this Mathew Williams and as Alice saw Mathew to the surgery, she suddenly remembered.

'You are the celebrity of the 11+ exam of a few years ago, aren't you?' said Alice excitedly.

'I'm sorry Mr Richardson, I just remembered that I saw Mr Williams on TV a few years ago. He was a huge celebrity then.

'Take a seat Mathew', said professor Richardson as his secretary closed the surgery door behind her.

'I have read your letter and was fascinated by your description of yourself and your brothers and would like to help you as much as I can.'

'Thank you very much professor for seeing me. What I would like to start with is to ask you, have you ever had any cases like me or should I say like the three of us?'

'The simple answer is no, but I am sure that it must be linked to the work carried out by the IVF clinics at the time you and your brothers were conceived.'

'I don't understand what are you referring to?'

'Well, I presume your mother was treated in a clinic possibly because she could not get pregnant in a normal way.'

'But I thought there are many children born after their mothers had received the IVF treatment!'

'Of course there are, but about fifteen, twenty years ago a small number of clinics tried to go further and there were many abortions, some of them induced, because of problems with the foetuses.

'By saying: "going further", do you mean using different methods?'

No, not that but trying to create methods to produce infants with predetermined characteristics.

'But how could it be possible that there are such huge differences in the abilities, bodies, minds and mental states of the three of us brothers.

To start with, we are triplets, which means we were affected equally with whatever was there in our mother's womb. Is it just a freak of nature or must there have been an interference by man?'

'Well, I'll give you an example' said professor Richardson.

'Some years ago a group of scientists, working for a pharmaceutical company, were investigating the possibility of dilating the arteries of the heart by oral treatment which would make presumably heart bypass unnecessary.

By oral treatment I mean prescribing medicine. There were some positive results with a number of volunteers but not enough. The sponsors and directors of these institutions were disappointed and the project on oral treatment of the heart arteries was stopped.

Few of the volunteers however stated in the questionnaire, relating to any side effects, that they felt a somewhat enhanced erection during the tests.

A few years later, with a new management, some of the company scientists remembered the volunteer's answers in their questioners and relayed this to the company board of directors and, the work was reactivated, but now, with the aim to improve the erection in men suffering from partial or total impotency.

What I mean to say is that when scientists carry out research in a particular field, it doesn't mean that the results will come, whether positive or negative, related to that field only. For example an undesired side-effect of synthetic chemicals released into the environment such as food chain may also be the ability to bind to hormone receptors and to block or activate them.'

'What effect would that have on pregnant mothers doctor?'

'Well, one defect could be that the sex of the baby would not be clear but, a cross over would occur like a male developing breasts at or after puberty.

It mostly depends on the type of chemicals influencing the development of the baby and, of course the quantity or, amount of chemicals introduced.

'Yes, I remember the thalidomide case were there were many physical malformations, but this is only one family and we are triplets.'

In your case, your mother and father could have been taking a number of different medicines and drugs before and during your mother's IVF treatment and some of, or a combination of, the chemicals taken contributed to the imbalance during the formation of the three fetal units.'

'Are there many cases like my family?'

'Well, up to about ten years ago, many clinics were using IVF methods and there are a number of children with small but detectable defects. At the time when your mother conceived, there was a race to create a designer baby by modifying the cells at the very start of conception'

Mathew was able to follow the analysis by the obstetrician but wanted to find out as much as possible from the renowned expert in the field that he, Mathew, has already read so much about.

'But why is it that my phallic and scrotal size, for example, is so large in relation to my overall body proportions.

Whatever effects there were, why would they be selective and affecting only some organs of the body? And why is one of my brothers almost twice the size of me and of our third brother?' asked Mathew.

'Well', said the doctor, ' if I could answer this, I would be a very wealthy man.

This is a very medical language I will use now Mathew:

It is well known in gynecology that in the prenatal male, in whom both the testicular and blood levels of testosterone are relatively low, testosterone is secreted and converted to 5alpha-dihydrotestosterone in the tissues possessing 5alpha-reductase. The low levels of this highly active androgen then exert local effects on the external genitalia, increasing phallic and scrotal size. This, so to say, creates normal human male, at least in that department. If it is possible to develop techniques to control the size and the contents of any part of our body chemically, or any other way, it is not to come in the near future. Today, medicine is fascinated with the thought of stem cells.

From your letter I could see that you read and know a great deal about this Mathew. Human development begins when a sperm fertilizes an egg and creates a single cell. This cell has a potential to form an entire organism. This cell is called totipotent cell. In the first 24 hours or so after fertilization, this cell divides and becomes, so called, conceptus.

If then the conceptus splits into two distinct groups of cells, it leads to a pregnancy with identical twins.

With ovulation and then fertilization of two eggs, or as we call them the oocytes, a double pregnancy occurs. In this case the twins are non-identical.

I believe that in your mother's case, two eggs were fertilized and created two separate cells and one of the cells, after becoming a conceptus, divided.

Without the interference of, I believe the chemicals, you and your brother Tom would have become identical twins.

As it is you differ in a number of points but for many people you are still identical. I mean in the appearance.

Now let me continue with the totipotent cells.

Approximately four days after the fertilization and after several cycles of division, these totipotent cells begin to specialize, forming a hollow sphere of cells, called a blastocyst. Inside the blastocyst is a cluster of cells that goes on to form virtually all the tissues of the human body. These cells are called pluripotent cells. They undergo further specialization into stem cells that are committed to give rise to cells that have a particular function.

For example blood stem cells give rise to red blood cells, white blood cells and platelets. They are called multipotent cells.

It is possible to influence the process I mentioned at

any stage by introducing various chemicals. The earlier one tries to influence the growth of a fertilized egg the greater is the damage, but to predict the outcome, we have to wait for a long time and even then I believe it will be a lottery were thousands would loose for one to gain.

There were rumours in the eighties and, nineties, of the last century that some medical laboratories here and in the United States were treating volunteers, men and women, promising the possibility of super babies, but this was denied by all the medical laboratories and the rumours, after some time, stopped.

If it was possible to control the cell division from totipotent to pluripotent and to stem cells by a single chemical element, appropriate research could last for years. The chemicals that influence cell divisions consist of many different atoms and molecules of different elements and the research using these would last many decades and even then, I do not believe, that the research would end there.'

'Thank, you professor Richardson, for seeing me. May I ask one more thing? If I find anything about my genetic parents' treatment, could I come again and see you please?'

'You must. I would like to know about it as much as you do.'

Mathew was, after this, even more confused than

before he met the professor. At night he would imagine that the time rushed back and the triplets were born again, this time with equal abilities and especially that they all stayed together with their mother and father.

On awakening he was so upset that work was the only cure to forget the events that made him the way he was now.

Now that the reunion was over, Claire and Mathew did not want to wait too long to get married and started planning straight away.

Mathew contacted David Bradshaw who now lived and worked in Birmingham and suggested a meeting. David and Mathew met for lunch in Birmingham and when Mathew asked David if he would be his best man at the wedding, David was over the moon.

'Mathew, my friend, that will be a treat for me. And if my mother is free could I bring her as well?'

'Of course. I'll be more than honoured.'

Mathew then contacted Mrs Paterson and said his fiancée Claire would like to ask her something. As Caroll was an adopted child herself, she understood Claire's desire and said she would be delighted to come.

Mathew was in two minds about asking Roger if he could give Claire away but Claire said she already asked him and his reply was it would be his pleasure and honour to do that.

Claire and Mathew did not want a church wedding. They both felt the ceremony in the registry office was sufficient. They did want a nice reception though and started planning it thoroughly. Actually it was Claire organizing the list. It was to consist of just over twenty people including themselves. Most will be Mathew's family and friends. Claire will have Caroll Paterson with her husband and Claire's three friends with partners.

Claire's friend Allison who has been her friend since the primary school, when hearing about the wedding, said:

'We know each other since we were children and I hope you want me to be your bridesmaid Claire.'

'Yes I do Allison, I wouldn't ask anybody else.'

When Mathew bought Claire the car for her birthday, they went for a drive and found themselves south of Shrewsbury on the A49.

After about 20 miles drive, they decided to have a meal to celebrate Claire's birthday and stopped at the Golden Arrow Hotel and it looked so attractive that they now decided to have the reception there.

Visiting the Hotel to organize the reception and make the reservation, they found the Hotel had changed. It looked even better after the refurbishment and the food was super as well.

The invitations were sent out and everybody invited was delighted to attend.

Geoff Martin wrote confirming his coming.

Last Saturday of June, Claire, we will be husband and wife, said Mathew stretching on the couch, his head on Clair's lap, Claire stroking his dark hair. He looked up and noticed Claire's face full of tears. He jumped up and sat beside her.

'What is it Claire, why the tears?'

'Oh Mathew. I'm so happy, I can't stop crying but I'm scarred as well.

'What are you scarred of Claire?'

'When I was younger, I dreamed of having my own place and sitting beside the man I love and I will soon have all that. Yet I'm scarred I will wake up from a dream and all this will disappear.

I am much older than you, Mathew, and one day you might find another, younger, girl and I will be alone again.

'Claire you know you are everything I have and everything I will ever want so wipe off your tears and let me whisper something in your ear!'

'Oh Mathew, my Mathew, this is the very first time you said that to me and I am sure it comes from your heart.'

Mathew did not have much contact with his brothers but did invite them to his and Claire's wedding.

Claire and Mathew invited Roger and Amanda for a meal and it couldn't have been better evening for the four of them. But it was Amanda who was in seventh haven. She liked Claire and her love for the home and her down to earth outlook on life.

Amanda was sad for them not to have a church wedding but at the same time delighted to have Mathew back and her face was blooming with happiness and she spent hours looking at the dresses and hats. Roger, on the other hand, could not forget Mathew's behavior when he lived with them, but was ecstatic with the change in his wife's health and happiness.

After the dinner was over, Mathew and Roger moved to the sitting room while Claire and Amanda stayed in the kitchen.

'Mathew, have you found out anything as to why were we told your mother died and all the other unexplained things?'

'Well, some. Our birth mother had IVF treatment but there must have been something else I need to find out, for example why would the clinic give my birth parents large sum of money to have the treatment when everybody else had to pay to have it done. Something does not add up.

I think there was some research involved and my birth parents signed certain papers prior to the treatment without even reading the agreement presented to them.

At that moment Amanda and Claire came in with coffee and apple pie Claire baked herself. When Roger tried the pie, it brought him back to his youth when his mother used to bake and the taste was just the same.

'Claire you are marvelous. I haven't enjoyed apple pie so much since I was ten years old. Mathew you are a lucky man!'

'I know dad. She is the best thing that happened to me.'

Roger pretended he was calm but inside he was boiling with feelings. Mathew had just called him dad again after all this time. He has matured and he has feelings after all and Amanda is glowing with happiness and looks ten years younger.

This was what Claire dreamed all through her growing up years, to have a family, to belong, to, love and be loved. And she had all this now.

'Claire are you all right. Is there something wrong dear?'

'No Mrs Williams. I am crying because I am so happy.'

The evening went better than anybody hoped for and when Roger and Amanda left, Claire gave Mathew a huge embrace and without a word the two of them went to the bedroom even forgetting to switch off the sitting room lights.

Amanda placed her head on Roger's shoulder as he started the car.

'Don't drive yet Roger. I want to enjoy this moment a little longer.'

'Amey, have you noticed anything different about Mathew?'

'Yes I did. He is very happy and I am delighted with everything and I think Claire is the best thing that could have happened to him.'

'I don't mean that. I mean, well, Mathew almost looks human. He even smiled tonight. That is first time ever I saw him actually smiling. I enjoyed tonight Amey. I really did.'

This meant more to Amey than if he said he loved her. She was like in a trance, feeling complete with peace and happiness in her heart.

'If this is the way their lives will proceed, than all the troubles and all the sad days she spent in her house thinking if she could have done it different, look minute comparing to the happiness that appears to be coming their family way.

The Wedding was set for July the 22nd in Shrewsbury registry office with the reception afterwards in the Golden Arrow Hotel on the A49 south of Shrewsbury.

It was only three weeks left and Claire was getting

very nervous. But Amanda was there to calm her down and help her getting everything in order. If anybody observed the two of them engrossed in activities like shopping or planning the reception details, they would think Amanda and Claire were mother and daughter.

At the registry office, besides Claire and Mathew, there were Roger and Amanda, David Bradshaw with his mother and Alison and her partner Jim Galloway.

'You look astonishing Claire', said Amanda, 'Mathew is a very lucky boy.'

'And I am very lucky to have him Mrs Williams.'

All those attending the wedding reception lived away from each other, every family traveled to the Golden Arrow Hotel in their own cars. Mathew and Claire had to have their own car as well as they were to start their honeymoon by driving to France.

At the arrival to the hotel, the adults met at the bar and Roger advised Mathew not to have any drinks before dinner and Mathew replied:

'Dad, I don't really enjoy alcohol, and I will do as you say with pleasure.'

While the starter was served, there were speeches by Roger, David, Geoff Martin and, of course, Mathew had to stand up and speak:

'I won't keep you from the food that is just arriving. Let me just say that I feel the happiest man on earth and my thanks for that first to my parents, then to David my best friend and pal, to Mr Martin who trusted me when I needed it and most of all to my wife Claire for coming into my life.'

Mathew sat down, looked at Claire and whispered: Was it all right what I said. I felt a bit dizzy and don't really recall what I said?'

'You were brilliant my husband.' Replied Claire with the smile.

Marion, the head waitress, made everybody feel at ease and the background music fitted perfectly with the murmur of the many conversations. But there was something she noticed or better something that wasn't there.

Although they were all supposed to be related, to one of the newlyweds, there was no warmth embracing the party as a whole but only existed separately within small groups of two or three people. It looked as if they met by accident and had nothing in common, thought Marion.

Once the dinner and the speeches were over Joe felt very tired and said to Ann he was going to have a rest. Paul and Ann booked two rooms and so did Irene for herself and Tom.

'What is wrong with Joe?' asked Paul when Joe left.

'He said he was a bit tired and went to have a short rest.' Answered Ann.

'My God, he is about the youngest and fittest person here. Is he getting lazy or what?'

But Ann did not hear Paul's comment. She recalled the words of the consultants about the approaching changes in Joe and was full of anxiety.

Tom kept himself to himself and stayed most of the time beside his mother.

'I don't think I will ever get married.' Tom whispered to Irene. 'I prefer to stay with you mum.'

The reception was over at about eleven and everybody came to Claire and Mathew to wish them many happy years together and asking them to reveal as to where they were going for their honeymoon, but it remained their secret.

Exactly at midnight the newlyweds said goodnight and withdrew to their room.

The wedding guests departed and the hotel staff started work to bring the reception room into a state suitable for another function.

Mathew calculated that the total journey to Carl Cambell was about 450 miles plus crossing from Portsmouth to St Malo in France and it would be nice to have an overnight break somewhere near St Malo. He looked at the "autoroute" on the internet and memorized the entire route from the Golden Arrow Hotel to the island of Olerona, a couple of weeks before the wedding.

Claire and Mathew had breakfast and drove off for their honeymoon at eight o'clock.

'Mathew, do you feel any closer to your brothers now, after you met them a few times. Tom looks quite like you although I can see that, besides the appearance, there is nothing else that links you to him.'

'No, not really, Claire. They are like any other people I meet. We have nothing in common, except that we are blood related, and I don't think we will ever get closer then to what we are now, but could you check that we have our tickets, money, passports and anything else you think we should have.'

'Yes master, everything is in order, you just take care and drive carefully.'

They drove from the Golden Arrow Hotel to the M54 and then joined the M40 south of Birmingham. Then Mathew decided to take the A34 and drove less fast round Oxford to Winchester and bypassing Southampton they arrived at Portsmouth's ferry port with enough time to spare.

The ferry journey was super. The see was calm and the crossing seemed as if the time stopped just for the two newlyweds.

Mathew made a few comments about the taste of the food they had, compared to Claire's home cooking but that was the only thing below top marks. After dark, they observed the rise of the full moon on the horizon and then retired to indulge in different pleasurable activities in their cabin.

In the morning they felt being on holidays for real. Having breakfast they saw in the distance the island of Jersey.

'Another few hours and we shall start driving on the right', said Claire but Mathew did not hear. He was already facing Carl Campbell and wondering what will he learn from the visit.

The first hundred miles, which was about half of the journey through France, was on the N137. It was very hot and they stopped a couple of times to refresh themselves with ice cream and then the journey took them closer to the Atlantic coast and driving was almost pleasant.

After driving round the city of Nantes there came the autostrade for about fifty miles but Mathew stayed on the road N137 and avoided paying the toll.

This road brought them past the town of La Rochelle and all the way to Rochefort.

From there, the journey took them through a few small towns and after crossing a bridge, they found themselves on the island Ile d'Orelon.

'Another twenty miles and we are there!' said Mathew and Claire opened her toilet bag to put some make up to her face.

'Mathew you are marvelous. Not a single wrong turning for the whole journey, as if you new where to go.'

'But I did. I memorized the journey and that was like being on the journey before.'

'May I speak to Mrs Williams please, my name is Irene Taylor.'

'She is out in the garden; I'll get her for you.'

Roger never heard of the name Taylor and wasn't sure he heard right so he just told Amanda there was a call for her.

'Yes, this is Amanda.'

'Hallo Amanda, this is Irene. I wonder if we could meet and have a chat concerning our boys.'

Yes, of course Irene, is there something concerning all three of them?'

'I am not sure. I talked to Ann and she would like to come as well.'

'Why don't you both come here for dinner and stay overnight. There is plenty of room for the both of you.'

Irene and Ann agreed and the visit was set for Saturday next. Roger was attending a conference and it was ideal for the three of them to have the weekend to themselves.

When Irene and Ann arrived there was quite a long spell of empty talk before Amanda broke the ice by asking

Irene about the anxiety she had when phoning her a few days ago.

'Our boys have something in common besides being brothers', started Irene. 'Each of them has a special field where he excels. Tom can remember music, Joe has extra strong physic and Mathew, as far as I understand visual memory.'

'But many people have a field where they are better than others. This is what makes us so different.'

'That is true, but I noticed that my Tom started loosing this gift and I took him to the specialist. They did a very thorough examination, which included the CT scan. They told me Tom might be aging much faster than a normal person would.

The consultants suggested another set of tests in twelve months time to do comparison', concluded Irene with a slight tremor in her voice.

'Oh my God' whispered Ann but audible enough to be heard by her two friends.

'Our Joe, as you saw, is a picture of health, but a while ago he complained having headaches when playing tennis. I too took him to the specialist in Chester and after doing some tests they organized a visit for us to a London clinic. When they compared the results from both clinics they suggested a possibility of early ageing of the body.'

'Well, so far I have not heard any of that from Mathew but I will have a talk with him without revealing anything we talked about here but could we keep all this among ourselves. If in time something comes up, we should meet again and have another talk. Do you agree?'

Irene opened her heart to the two friends and talked about her husband leaving and how it affected Tom. Amanda felt much better when she was able to come out about Mathew leaving home after he found out about being adopted and how everything was smoothed when he discovered they were honest with him all the time.

Ann talked of Paul's and her disappointment when Joe, aged five, showed such a low IQ and relief when they realized he was so good in the game of tennis.

Now all the fears from the past have reappeared although in different form.

Roger phoned and Amanda was delighted to tell him she is enjoying herself having her two friends staying over-night.

Amanda served the dinner and after a glass of vine, the three mothers got even closer to each other. They chatted well into the night. When Amanda closed her bedroom door and started getting ready for bed she started praying.

At first it was just her thoughts and whisper. Then she knelt beside her bed and closed her eyes. She saw

Mathew with Claire and a little baby, sitting in her back garden happily enjoying the spring sun. But when she came closer to them Amanda noticed that her Mathew looked very old and she started to cry.

'Please God, Mathew is a very nice boy. He has suffered so much, he deserves some happiness. Let him enjoy a little longer now that he has found happiness with Claire who is such a nice girl. I love her as if she was my daughter.'

But the image of Mathew she saw in the garden would not go away and in the morning she had to work on her face in order to hide the sleepless night.

The three mothers decided to stay in contact and relay any changes in their children but keep all that to themselves.

'Hello Mr Campbell, I am Mathew, Mike Osborne's son, and this is my wife Claire.'

'Hello Mathew, come in please, come in. It has been so hot this week, we keep the doors shut and the air conditioning on.'

'Ida, these are our visitors Claire and Mathew, and this is my wife Ida.'

'Take a seat please, you must be tired driving in this heat.' Said Carl's wife and started pouring fresh orange juice for the four of them.

'From your letter I understood this is your first trip abroad. Was it difficult to find us?'

'Mathew memorized the whole journey and drove as if he had been here many times before.' Added Claire.

'Are you both working back home?'

'Yes we are. I do temping and Mathew has his own show and is involved in research at the university', said Claire with pride.

'What is temping', asked Ida.

'I do secretarial work but am self employed. I get jobs with different companies through secretarial agencies.

'Ah yes like locum doctors here. They temporary replace family doctors, no', added Ida.

'Looking at you and thinking back, your hair and your eyes are your dad's but nothing else as far as I can remember.'

'Claire could you help me in the kitchen and let the two of them have a chat.'

'Of course Mrs Campbell, you have a beautiful house and the island is like a paradise with so much green and no big buildings around.'

It really was like heaven on earth with houses, with their red roofs and white walls, set well behind their front gardens, full of flowers between the green foliage of the shrubs and trees.

'Mathew, when you phoned, I was really surprised to

hear Sharon's children were declared dead to her and their mother was declared dead to the families that adopted them, so I have been putting my thoughts to paper and I hope this may help answer some of your questions so can we start with this:

When Sharon was about a couple of months pregnant, the clinic suggested abortion saying there were complications, but Sharon was adamant to see the pregnancy through and contacted me and I was able to scare the clinic.

They agreed for the pregnancy to continue although they were to supply the doctor to oversee the pregnancy to the end. Soon after that my family was struck with tragedy, my wife and daughter were killed in a traffic accident and I was very depressed for some time.

I remember writing a letter to your mother giving her the sad news and informing her about my move to France or at least about selling the business and that is about all I could think about.'

'Yes, my mother never opened the letter you sent her. I found it a few months ago in her suitcase in the hospital where she is still a patient. Do you recall anything about the clinic my mother had the IVF treatment in?'

'I do. The Clinic was called The First English American Medical Services. I remember the official Clinic letter with the abbreviation FEAMS. It was located just outside the village of Studley off the A435 about 15 miles south of Birmingham. As far as I remember it stayed open for about three to four years. As far as I know your mother was the only one giving birth after getting the IVF treatment, where the children lived for more than two years.

'What was the reason for that Mr Campbell, were there only very few women treated or was the success rate so low?'

'Neither. Some women were told the pregnancy went wrong and some were given more money to agree to terminate their pregnancies. After three or four years or so the Clinic simply disappeared.'

'Carl could you talk to Mathew and Claire and persuade them that we want them to stay with us, at least for a few nights' said Ida bringing the food which filled the sitting room with delicious smell.

'I wouldn't have it any other way. You are actually the very first English visitors here and I was your father's best man, all those years ago.'

'So it's settled then. Claire let us bring your luggage to your room ant Mathew and Carl could have another chat. Carl, Claire and I will go for a short walk. We'll be out for about an hour', and it is the best way for you to give Mathew as much time as possible to ask anything he needed answers to.

'Mr Campbell, I found a slip indicating payment

of twenty five thousand pounds to my parents account through The First New York Bank. Could that help in tracing any of the people in charge of the Clinic some nineteen years ago?'

'Well, if that is all there is, I am not sure. Is there anything else you can find Mathew?'

'Maybe I can. I visited my birth mother, Sharon, on my own and took all papers I could find in her suitcase but have not studied yet the bits and pieces she had.'

'It would be worth seeing what you have and then see what could be done. But what is your intention, just curiosity or to confront the people and doctors that ran the Clinic?'

'I don't have enough details, of what happened, to be able to give an answer now. Could I seek your advise when I sort out all I could Mr Campbell?'

'Of course Mathew but we have done enough for today. Let me show you my garden where I spend most of my time these days.'

'You know Ida is my second wife. As I told you I lost my first wife and daughter in a traffic accident and Ida's husband died about the same time almost at the same spot when the two of them were holidaying in England. They had no children and I was asked to represent her in court. I was too upset and had a few weeks off but did meet Ida later and after about eighteen months we met again and we started correspondence and the result was that after a couple of years we got married.

This garden is my baby. It was just a piece of land when we came here and I spent a lot of time and effort to make it as it looks today. It gives me peace and tranquility.'

'Are these real oranges Mr Campbell?'

'They are. All the fruit you see is edible and Ida makes loads of jam every autumn.'

'Ah there you are. Claire and I will set the table and give you a call soon. The young ones must be starving.'

It was like being on a different planet. The walk through the little town, after breakfast, wearing just a tee shirt, shorts and sandals and of course sunglasses was superior in every way to anything Claire experienced in her life, holding Mathew's hand and glowing with happiness.

'I am delighted Mathew and Claire are staying for another couple of days', said Ida to her husband. 'Even you look happier as if they injected some extra life into you.'

'Yes they did. It is nice to have young ones around the house even if it is for a few days only.'

When the young ones returned the Campbells took them for a slow drive around the island and showed them the many beaches.

They had lunch at a small cafe and returned to the house early afternoon and Ida excused herself and went for the afternoon rest.

'What sort of show do you have Mathew if I may ask.'

'Of course Mr Campbell. I have the ability to memorize a very large amount of data and people come to the show writing down their particulars which I scan just once and then I can give back any of the data to any of the say fifteen hundred people. And I get paid for that.'

'But how much data do you need to remember in order for the show to be a success?'

'Well about fifteen to twenty thousand bits of information', said Mathew modestly.

'And how often do you have such shows Mathew?'

'Almost every Saturday for the last two and half years.'

'My God', whispered Carl. 'You couldn't have inherited that from your parents. Mike could not remember what hole he was playing, if asked, when we used to play golf, and your mother, although working with figures, never knew how much she paid for when she came back from her shopping.'

'Were they very happy together?'

'They behaved as if they were courting, always together and always happy. I remember Mike saying to a couple having difficulty with their marriage to pretend not to be married and you know Mathew, it worked.'

'What happened when he developed the heart problem?'

'Yes, that was hard to take. First he did not believe it was permanent and saw three different consultants but they all gave the same diagnosis. But Mike was a fighter and accepted that his life had to change and he was fine. Then the accident happened with the lorry coming from nowhere and it was so tragic seeing Sharon in hospital, pregnant but without Mike to give her his support.'

'Mr Campbell, I shall go through the papers my birth mother had and will send you copies of what I think are important ones for me. I would be thankful if you could look through and possibly advise me as to what else I could do.

I visited your old offices, as you know, and was going to ask Mr Tompkins if he could represent me but I would like very much if you would agree to do that, but charging your usual fees as Claire and I wouldn't have it any other way.'

'Mathew dear I am retired and do not take paid work any more but I'll make an exception and take your case if there comes the need for it. But it might need a detective to prod deeper because, as far as I remember, the Clinic and the staff working in it were very secretive.

Very little was known while it was open and accepting patients. I will, if that is all right with you, consult a friend of mine who is by now retired but was a detective all his working life and I'll let you know what could be done either by me or involving my friend as well.'

Mathew did not ask any more questions. He was convinced now that his parents were like any other; a normal couple trying to get on in life and loving each other. He imagined the building of the Clinic where the IVF treatment took place and the doctors involved as evil people doing experiments with people whom they were supposed to help.

Claire and Mathew invited the Campbells for an evening meal and thanked them for their hospitality. Next morning they said farewell and Ida embraced Mathew and Claire as if they were part of her family.

'Take care on the road and this house is always open if you feel like coming to visit us for a holiday. We really enjoyed your company.'

Carl and Ida watched them driving off and waved till the car turned left onto the main island road and disappeared from view. Carl noticed tears in Ida's eyes but said nothing. He felt just like she did, they had "their children" with them for a few days and felt emptiness at their departures.

'We'll see them again Ida. If not here then in England,

as I am sure Mathew will want me to take up the case he is looking into.'

As the young ones drove over the bridge leaving the island of Oleron Claire spoke with her eyes closed:

'Mathew, it was like being at home and on holidays at the same time.

I really enjoyed the last four days.'

'They are nice, aren't they, said Mathew. 'We must send them a nice present when we come home, will you see to that Claire, you are much better at it than I am.'

Mathew drove through a few villages and when they came to within a few miles from Rochefort Mathew had the toll money available so not to disturb Claire who was sound asleep. Driving past Rochefort they were to join the N137 for La Rochelle. At the roundabout Mathew suddenly felt strange. He did not recognize the road he had memorized in detail before starting their holidays.

At the first parking sign he stopped and took out the road map but it wasn't of much use, as he did not know where they were to start with. He could not recall the memorized details and the more he tried, the more frustrated he became. There was very little traffic and the quietness made Claire wake up. She opened her eyes and noticed the expression of fear on Mathew's face.

'What is it Mathew, is the car all right?'

'Claire I don't know where we are. I must have taken

a wrong turning somewhere and I do not recognize this road.'

'It's not the end of the world Mathew. It could happen to anybody. Let us have a sandwich and a cold drink and then we will decide what to do.'

Claire noticed some kind of panic in Mathew's behavior and wanted to calm him down. As she unwrapped the sandwiches the sun came out from behind the lonely cloud and Claire noticed that it was on their left side.

'Shouldn't the sun be on our right in the morning Mathew if we are traveling north?'

This was an impulse for Mathew's brain to start reasoning.

'Of course it should be. You are a genius Claire. We will turn around and watch for the road signs. Here, you keep the road map and try to find out where we are.'

'Mathew did we pass the toll place marked here?'

'Yes we did about ten miles ago.'

'Then we must be somewhere between the toll place and Rochefort, I think.'

Mathew was relieved, by passing on the responsibility to Claire and Claire very quickly noticed the sign for Rochefort and La Rochelle.

'There is a roundabout ahead Mathew. We are taking the third exit on the right.'

'How strange. I can't remember being here yet I must

have come and taken a wrong exit and drove back south. But I have a first class navigator and we cannot go wrong now.'

It was the second time since Claire met Mathew that he forgot anything. The first time was when he left his mobile phone off after the police talked to him at Mr Martin's office and now this. But this one worried her because of the way it affected her man.

Claire directed Mathew to the N137 road and by-passing the town of La Rochelle they continued on the same road number until they reached the autostrade A83 which brought them to Nantes where Claire directed Mathew to the road N137 again and towards the town of Rennes. Just before Rennes they decided to stop and have lunch.

Mathew was back in his old form. He looked relaxed and ate well and when Claire asked him if he recognizes the road he said:

'Of course I do, why shouldn't I?'

Claire said nothing but the worry stayed with her for the rest of the journey.

They reached the ferry terminal at St Malo and after boarding and getting the cabin for the night Claire forgot all about the journey and the two of them enjoyed another romantic evening on the deck of the ferry.

Soon after reaching the island of Jersey the weather

changed. It got cold and they retired to their cabin. It was the first night since they started living together that they fell asleep without making love. Actually Claire pretended to have fallen asleep but her thoughts of the past day were back with her.

Next morning Mathew was full of himself and the journey from Portsmouth home was very pleasant. They bypassed Southampton driving on the M37, joined A33 and at Winchester took A34 all the way to Birmingham. Using the motorway ring road and M54 and finally A5, they reached Shrewsbury, their hometown.

Coming to the front door of their flat, Mathew remembered to carry Claire inside and jokingly said:

'Don't you get any heavier or I won't be able to do this again.'

By the time Mathew brought the cases upstairs and Claire set up the table with two cups of tea and a cake she defrosted, it was nine o'clock and she decided to phone Roger and Amanda.

'Hello Mrs Williams, this is Claire. We have come back just this minute. Yes it was wonderful thank you. I might be able to come and visit you tomorrow if that is fine with you but here is Mathew, he wants to talk to you as well.'

'Hello mum. Yes we did. We had a lively time. I am

at the University of Wrexham tomorrow but will come soon to see you and dad.'

Amanda was in seventh heaven. She forgot all the talk about something being not right with the boys and was looking forward to see her daughter in law to hear all the news about their honeymoon.

Sitting down with Roger, Amanda said:

'Roger, do you think we might become grandparents soon? But Roger didn't mind one way or the other as long as his wife was happy.

When Claire came through the door she was glowing with happiness and Amanda could not resist giving her a long tight hug.

'Come in dear, come in. Roger is out and it will give us time to chat as daughter and mother because you are more than that to me. Tell me where did you go, we all wondered but nobody could guess.'

Well, we drove to France and for the last four days stayed with Mr and Mrs Campbell.

Carl Campbell was a school friend of Mathew's real dad and he wanted to ask him what he new about the time before Mathew was born, or something like that.'

'Did you share the driving. Mathew sounded a bit tired when we talked to me last night?'

'He drove there and back. It was easier that way as Mathew remembered all the roads there and back. He just made one slip on the whole journey and that really shocked him.'

'What do you mean shocked, was it a traffic accident or something dangerous?'

'I'm not sure. I was asleep and when I woke up the car was parked and Mathew just sat there not knowing what to do. I was really worried about him you know because he is always sure. Once he remembers he never forgets but this time he did.'

Amanda remembered her talk with Irene and Anna and felt goose pimples all over her body. She did not dare to mention that to Claire and said:

'Maybe he ate something. Sometimes it makes you dumb although you don't feel as if your stomach is upset at all.'

'Yes, I shouldn't worry. But he did look as if he was lost. It might had lasted for a short time only but I hope it was as you said, the food.'

'Claire darling, you know I love Mathew and I love you as much and if ever anything comes you would like to talk about I will be always here for both of you, you know that.'

'I know Mrs Williams and I love you as if you were my mother. Please don't mention to Mathew I was worried about him. It was probably nothing and there is no point worrying him.'

Late that day when Mathew came home from Wrexham University he was back to his normal behaviour. They had dinner and he explained to Claire that the University research group would like to extend the project for further three years and will send him their proposal within a few weeks. They celebrated with a few sips of schnapps and a glass of wine and on Claire's suggestion they went for a short walk. Before going to bed, Mathew had a shower and in bed, Claire felt, he was stronger than his usual not that she ever complained.

On the contrary, it made her completely forget the event that happened on the road in France after leaving the Campbells.

The letter from the Wrexham University arrived as expected and Mathew was delighted with the offer and the amount of time he would be engaged there. He enjoyed the company of the research students and Professor Horowitz. Although there was another year of the first agreement to run it appeared that the University group were keen to have Mathew for themselves and not to lose him to some other university.

There was added information by professor Horowitz that instead of the increase in payment the university would include him into the university insurance scheme starting with this year's autumn term. Mathew decided to phone professor Horowitz and ask what would that entail and was told that the insurance scheme covers graduated pension premiums loss of earnings in case he, Mathew, would not, for any reason, be able to perform using his memorizing ability and health benefits.

'Claire was as happy as a young bride could be. She cuddled beside her husband and scanned over the pages of the agreement Mathew was holding in his hands and noticed the offer of the insurance. The memory of the event on the French road came back to her and she asked Mathew.

'What do they mean by offering you the insurance Mathew, is it dangerous what you do there?'

'No Claire. I think they are not able to offer me more money and they think the insurance would seem as an extra. But I am delighted because I like it there and it is only two days a week and only during the university term time which makes it thirty weeks a year. Not bad for somebody that left school at the age of fifteen. What do you say Claire?'

'I love you my husband but don't forget we are dining with your parents tonight. We have half an hour to get ready.'

Mathew became attached to his adopted parents since he and Claire decided to get married. It was something he never thought could happen. They were so pleasant and showed their delight seeing him and Claire married and happy.

Roger and Amanda, on the other hand, saw Mathew a very changed man from what he was as a child and teenager. He was pleasant, considered and showed respect and love towards her and Roger. Yes, Amanda was sure it was love and she glowed with happiness. Now and then she would remember the meeting she had with Irene and Anna but seeing her son so happy and full of joy, the thoughts dispersed and her face radiated happiness again.

'Roger I am so happy Mathew and Claire are coming tonight. It is... But before she could finish what she wanted to say, Roger came to her and gave a tight hug. 'It is nice to have a family, isn't it Amy?'

'That was exactly what I was going to say. I hope nothing changes for a very long time.'

Claire and Mathew came about six and there were no hesitations but honest greetings and the questions started straight away about the honeymoon and the journey through France.

Roger was so much at ease that he simply sat beside Claire with his arm around her shoulders listening to Mathew's chat with Amanda as if it has always been that way. Claire looked at Roger but she could not read his thoughts.

She did not know how low the relations between Mathew and his adopted parents dropped, culminating with Mathew's departure and Amanda's depression periods. These last few months have been like one miracle after another and Amanda looked fulfilled and as happy as a young girl in love.

'Claire the dinner is ready but it is a bit early to sit down. Shall we go for a stroll and let these two men have a chat without the two of us interfering.

Roger, we will be back in half an hour but don't drink too much as I made a large meal and it is something you and Mathew used to like very much.'

At the departure of Amanda and Claire, Mathew sat facing Roger and Said:

'Dad may I ask you something?'

'Of course Mathew, fire away!'

'You know how I make my money using my memory. Well on our journey back through France, while Claire was asleep, I suddenly couldn't say where I was so I stopped at the first parking place and tried to sort myself out but I just did not know what had happened and where on the road map were we.'

'It happens to me many times son. It is nothing special and nothing to worry about.'

'I was really scarred you know. Thanks to Claire who

reasoned with me, we, or better Claire, sorted the mistake and got us on our way again.'

After a pause Roger said that professor Horowitz mentioned a second contract he offered to Mathew and how he was delighted with the results so far.

Roger showed real interest in the work Mathew did with the Wrexham University and Mathew felt his father was proud of him.

'You know dad I wish I could have been different when I lived here. As if there was something wrong with me I had no feelings for you, mum and as a matter of fact for anybody else.

Not that I was selfish or trying to justify myself, no. I think the IVF treatment my birth mother was receiving contributed a lot. Even my two brothers have problems mixing with other people.'

At that moment Amanda and Claire entered and in no time the dinner was served.

'You young ones should not drive back tonight, so you may have another drink if you feel like having one', said Amanda.

The two of them looked at each other and decided to stay for the night.

Claire woke up, put the bedside light on and noticed it was only half past two. Mathew appeared to be in some kind of discomfort, covered with sweat and making sounds as if arguing with somebody.

'Mathew, darling, are you all right. Would you like a glass of water?'

Claire noticed his facial expression was just like she saw when he lost his way on the French road five days previously. He had two glasses of wine the night before they left the Campbells and he had wine last night. But he had wine before and did not upset him. She remembered they had wine the day they made love for the very first time and it did not upset Mathew one bit, on the contrary....

'Maybe there was something in the wine', thought Claire and went to the bathroom to wet the towel and wipe Mathew's face and body as he was covered with sweat.

'Claire I had a bad dream. I was shut in a tiny room and the walls were shouting at me saying I was adopted but was not wanted and will stay alone all my life.

Then a lot of dead bodies appeared around me and the voice came back shouting that these are my only relatives and that I will never be loved. It was horrible I tell you.'

'It's fine now Mathew, you know that is not true and we all love you.'

Claire put Mathew's head on her shoulder and he fell asleep with his arm on her chest.

'Did last night's dinner agree with you two?', asked Amanda in the morning, remembering she heard the two young ones talking and going to the bathroom in the middle of the night.

'It was ten out of ten', said Claire and Mathew agreed: 'Your dinners always taste good mum.'

Roger phoned his office saying he was not coming to work for the day and enjoyed the expression of happiness on Amanda's face.

The house felt like a real home, worm, pleasant, comfortable…. If he had a button on his computer to stop the time he would have done it without any hesitation. He would have stopped it forever.

He went to the kitchen, returning his cup and saucer where Amanda and Claire were doing tidying up and said to Amanda:

'I love you, my angel.'

Claire blushed and when Roger left she asked:

'Is he always like this?'

'Roger is sweet and thoughtful man but when Mathew left home he became a loner, a recluse. All the fun had drained out of him and then I became ill and, well, we went through a difficult period Claire but now both of us are as happy as little children. And Mathew couldn't have found a better wife if he looked for a thousand years.

'Hello Irene, this is Amanda.'

'Amanda dear, I was just thinking about you. I got a recipe for "lasagne al forno" but, when served, Tom and I did not like it at all. I wonder what I did wrong?'

'If you would like I could come and we can give it a try together and we could invite Anna and have another chat, just the three of us.'

'Oh that would be marvelous, tell me what days would suit you and I can sort it out with Anna?'

'Any day really, Irene. I could bring a few photographs of Mathew's and Claire's honeymoon. They went to France and had a wonderful time.'

The getting together for the three mothers was arranged and Amanda was to stay overnight at Irene's in Cranspole.

Tom and Irene were looking at the family photographs and when he saw the photo of the reunion taken just over a year previously, he was amazed that he could be in two places in one photograph.

'No Tom, this is you and that is your twin brother Mathew. It was the very first time the three of you met since you were born.'

'Oh yes I remember', said Tom but he only said that in order not to worry his mother.

There were patches of loss in his memory, which he accepted uncomplainingly as part of his attitude to the changes in his life. Although the childhood was startlingly vivid, recent events have been mislaid or, worse, misplaced. The selfishness of the father, the adopted father that is, which left a discomfort in his memory and he never wanted to see him again, was as fresh as it could be. On the other hand Tom could be seeing a music title and listening to the music at the same time, and not recognizing that the two were in any way connected.

Anything Irene read about the tonic in memory enhance-ment, she introduced to Tom's diet. Green vegetables, green salads including sage and parsley was on the menu daily and she tried to convince herself that Tom's condition was not deteriorating as fast as it would had been otherwise.

Amanda heard from Claire how Mathew became worried driving back through France and when Roger told her that Mathew mentioned the incident to him as well, she decided to reveal this to Irene and Anna when they meet.

The three mothers embraced each other and while Irene went to the drink cabinet to pour them a drink, Amanda started talking about their son's reunion and after a few details were remembered, the silence fell upon the three of them.

Amanda was the first to speak, and there was a mixture of sadness and fear in her voice.

'I think our Mathew is not well, that's why I wanted us to meet.

Maybe I am only imagining but one thing that Mathew's had in him, good memory, appears to be affected.' And Amanda's eyes filled with tears.

'I pray and hope I'm wrong but the fear would not go away.'

'Amanda', said Irene: Mathew and Tom are identical twins and I noticed similar thing with Tom. As you know he could learn to play the piano simply by listening to me playing. In fact he learnt only by listening, but lately I noticed he has been having difficulty recalling things he learned within the last year, although anything that happened years ago is still fresh in his mind. He had a CT scan and they, the doctors, wanted him to have another one a year later. They said his brain is ageing prematurely.'

There was a long spell of silence and then Ann spoke:

'My son Joe doesn't have much in his head to worry about but I'm afraid he is getting old physically. I took him for a check up and was told that Joe will age quicker than normal. I don't really understand what it means except that the only thing he could do, to play tennis, is getting too hard for him.

This time the silence was hurting.

'Why, why is it happening to our boys? Could this have been inherited or have we done something to trigger it?' Whispered Amanda, scared now even more when she heard about the other two boys with similar problems.

'What about the three of us taking our boys to the clinic I took Tom a few months ago and, let the doctors compare the results of the tests on all of them.

Maybe it would help the doctors find out what are the reasons for this illness or whatever they call it', suggested Irene and waited for the answers.

Ann was the first of the two mothers to agree and then Amanda, her eyes full of tears, just nodded.

The hardest thing, to open their hearts to each other, was the first step of many the mothers were to take. Apprehension and not knowing what was the next step going to demand from each or all three of them increased their fear.

They decided to make an appointment with their appropriate consultants and present them with the state of health of the other two of the triplet brothers and suggest that the three have a medical, based on their up to date medical test results.

This way, if there is any way to turn around the deterioration or at least stop it, it might be found before it becomes too late.

On her way home, Amanda realized that she needed to talk to Claire. In fact she should have talked to her daughter in law before going to meet Ann and Irene but, fearing for her son, she completely forgot Mathew's wife.

Claire was actually in a desperate state. She could not talk to her husband and express her fears and Mathew's parents, especially Amanda, were in a similar state as herself.

Then she remembered Carl. He mentioned, when Claire and Mathew visited him in France, that, if required, he would be willing to get involved although he did mention that an investigation by a professional detective would help.

Mathew was not able to continue with his Saturday shows but his contract with the University was to continued for some time still.

On the day he went to Wrexham University, Claire sat down determined to write and ask Carl Campbell for help.

Dear Mr Campbell,

I hope you and Mrs Campbell are well .

I am writing this letter without consulting with Mathew

as I am very worried and scared concerning his state of health.

Mathew was never strong physically and his ability to use his extraordinary memory made him believe in himself. But since we came back from visiting you, Mathew has been going down steadily. He has aged and looks almost twice the age he is and his memory has been affected as well. He, often, could not remember recent events, even very simple ones. Anything that happened more than a year ago he can still manage but, that does not help him with his work and he had to give it up.

I pray that maybe if it could be possible to find what happened to him before he was born, there might be a chance to find a medicine that would make my Mathew well again.

You mentioned, when Mathew and I were visiting your home, that there was a special clinic.

If there is anything that you may be able to do, Mathew and I would be grateful for ever.

Yours,

Claire

She addressed the letter and took it to the post office to get a correct stamp but, as soon as she placed the letter into the mail box, she got scared.

Claire walked home in confusion and fear. She saw Carl finding the details taken down by the doctors during

Sharon's IVF treatment and subsequent pregnancy tests results telling her that her man, her lover and everything she has had, was infected with a decease that could not be treated. Her eyes were full of tears when a man grabbed her as she was crossing the street.

'Are you all right dear, you almost went under that lorry?'

As she came back from her thoughts, Claire noticed she was in the middle of the street just a couple of feet in front of a lorry and a number of people, with their faces showing concern.

Amanda decided to invite Claire for a chat by suggesting she needed help and advice with shopping for herself.

As Claire was not working full time but as a temp, she chose the day when Mathew was at the University. Amanda agreed as for her any day, the sooner the better would be fine .

'I would like that Mrs Williams. I was actually thinking to ask you if the two of us could meet and have a talk. I'll be at your house early afternoon.'

Claire noticed Mathew's problem more than anybody else. She noticed Mathew putting his coat on and then going to the bathroom.

Above the ears on her husband's head, Claire could see grey hair appearing and squirting his eyes when a print was somewhat smaller or if the light was not sufficiently bright. But the main worry was his memory. As long as her man could work, and the only work he was able to do was using his memory, he could look forward to it. If this was taken away from Mathew, it would be a big blow for him.

Before coming to her mother in law's house, Claire tried to look as if all is well but could not last for long.

As soon as Amanda brought her into the sitting room and said:

'Claire, my dear, I would like us to have a talk about Mathew', she went numb and her eyes filled with tears.

Amanda got scared thinking she did something wrong but Claire looked at her mother in law and whispered:

'I am scared too Mrs Williams. Mathew is everything I have and everything I ever wanted but I am scared there is something happening to my husband. He has become very forgetful.

Anything that happened a year ago or more, he can recall with a bit of effort but, he started to forget the details that happened recently. I thought it was him being overworked but I fear his memory is fading.'

Amanda gave Claire a hug and held her tight.

'Claire, dear, I talked to Irene and Ann last Saturday. There is something happening to Mathew's brothers as well and I wonder if there is a link.

We talked about taking the three of them to a specialist clinic in London to see if they could diagnose either individually or find if there is a connection. But you are Mathew's wife and it has to be up to you to decide.'

As Amanda looked at Claire, she noticed her daughter in law's face pale and wet with tears. First thing coming to her mind was that Claire might be pregnant but, seeing sad and desperate face, she just gave Claire a hug and waited for a response from Claire and after a while it came.

'Mrs Williams, I am desperately worried for Mathew. I even wrote a letter to Mr Campbell, without Mathew knowing of course, to see if there is anything he could find from the clinic the brothers were conceived in, something that could give the doctors now an indication as to how to treat their condition. I just posted the letter a few days ago.

'I am so glad you were able to come my friend', Carl Campbell greeted Marcelo at the Angouleme airport, about seventy miles from his house.

'How was the journey Tania?', Carl asked Marcelo's wife as he greeted her with a hug.

'It was not as long as traveling by car Carl; and how is Ida?'

'She is at home looking forward to having you both.'

Carl and Ida had, a couple of years previously, befriended Marcelo and his wife Tania during their holidays on the island of Krk in Croatia where Tania and Marcelo have their home.

Carl and his wife Ida rented a small boat and, although advised by the boat owner not to leave the bay as the weather was worsening and a strong northerly wind could affect the small boat, they forgot about the danger and enjoyed their afternoon sightseeing the neighboring beaches. By the time the wind picked up strength they were too far to be able to return safely with the four horse power outboard motor.

Marcelo was out there fishing and was ready to return to the bay suspecting imminent strengthening of the north wind, when he noticed a small boat in trouble.

He offered his help and brought them safely back. They became friends and the two couples spent a number of evenings together.

Carl and Ida were so grateful, they invited their friends to visit them in France and this was it.

It took Carl less than two hours of slow driving and there was Ida at the door welcoming their visitors and friends.

'Hello Tania, come in please and our hero Marcelo.

You will, I am sure, have an espresso before anything else.'

While Ida and Tania went to the kitchen, Carl and Marcelo talked boats and fishing. Then Carl said:

Marcelo I have a very sad case you might want to help with.

And Carl brought a file from his desk.

Marcelo studied the notes Carl placed in front of him and after a while responded:

'Carl this sounds like happening a hundred years in the future and not now.

I can't imagine experiments like these had or will ever bee performed. It was totally inhumane.'

'Marcelo, you told me you intend to visit your friends in England. Could I persuade you to join me and the youngsters affected by these experiments, to spend a day or two and see if you have any idea as to how to proceed in finding as much as possible who the culprits were and where they are now.

They might be still repeating their experiments some-where else on the innocent unsuspecting couples.'

'Of course my friend. Tania will be glad she could have a day browsing through the shops in London with her friend Beth without me nudging her to move on.

After spending a few pleasant day with their friends, Marcelo and Tania were taken by Carl to the local airport from where they flew directly to Southampton airport in England. There was a fast train taking them to London Paddington station where they were met by their friend John Higgins.

'Welcome Marcelo, Tania! This is the best time to arrive, especially it being Saturday, as there are no traffic jams and our car journey will be quite short. Beth is looking forward to you coming and has already made plans to take you Tania out as much as you can take, so prepare yourself for the worst.'

Marcelo felt as if he was driving the car, sitting on the front passenger seat and his body jerked at every manoeuvre the car made on their journey to the Higgins household.

'You mentioned you might have to travel up north helping a friend. Is that on police business or something else?

'It might be. I'm not sure yet if I could be of any help but I promised my friends in France I will try. It involves a sad case, 20 years old and I could not say no to their plea.

Marcelo and Tania enjoyed their hosts company for the rest of the day and the following day, Sunday.

On Monday morning Marcelo took a local bus that took him to Victoria Coach Station in London where he purchased a ticket to Birmingham.

He traveled from London by coach. Leaving Victoria coach station at seven thirty the traffic was not as bad as he was told it would be later on in the morning but even so it took them a while to get out of London. Once on the motorway M40, the coach speed appeared, what Marcelo guessed, a constant seventy mph. One and a half hours later, the coach entered the Birmingham bus terminal where Marcelo was met by Carl and, what Marcelo thought from reading Carl's notes, young Mathew and his wife Claire.

Claire looked like a young lady in her mid twenties but Mathew appeared as a worn out and frail, aged teenager.

After exchanging greetings and introductions Marcelo was asked if he would like a snack and they could have a chat.

From the bits of information Mathew took from his mother's suitcase there was very little extra that could help, Marcelo thought but at least, the details on the cheque receipt could link the Clinic to the Osborne family.

'Would it be possible to visit your mother, Mathew, your birth mother that is?'

Mathew was looking slightly confused and Carl interrupted by saying it is the first thing on the agenda for the morning and after finishing paying the waitress, the four left to visit Sharon Osborne.

Coming to the garden bench Sharon was sitting on, she recognized Mathew and then had a very long stare at Carl. Slowly her face changed from fear to curiosity and finally to delight.

'Carl, is that you? You have changed. When they told me I was going to have visitors today, I thought Mike was coming and then I remembered that he died but I could not remember how long ago. But I am glad you came to see me.'

'Sharon this is a very good friend of mine Marcelo.'

'What a strange name. Where does it come from?'

'Mrs Osborne, when you were in the hospital expecting your baby, were there many mothers like you there?'

'You mean pregnant. There were three rooms in the Clinic with beds and there were three beds in each room, sometimes only two.'

'And where they kept the new born babies? Beside mothers beds or elsewhere?'

'Oh no. I have never seen a baby in the Clinic. There were no babies born while I was there. You see we were told that we were all very difficult cases and many pregnancies terminated within two to three months from conception and that that was why there were no babies in the Clinic. But my husband and I had a very good layer and I was allowed to give birth but was told that, unfortunately, my babies died at birth. That was the cause of my illness that lasted for a very long time. Carl could tell you how long as I am not so sure.'

'Sharon Osborne was, by now, very sleepy and there was no point to continue with questions and Marcelo and Claire went out leaving Carl and Mathew to have a few private moments with Sharon.

Next they drove to where the original Clinic, the FEAMS was located.

'This is the building that used to be the so called The First English American Medical Services or FEAMS as it was called', explained Carl after the four of them got out of the car.

'The outside of the building probably looks the same and the car park is still here although not as tidy as it used to be I presume.'

There were a number of skips some of them full to the top, crying to be taken away, placed there recently and waiting to be filled.

Walking towards the main entrance, Marcelo noticed a large amount of electronic gear in two skips.

'Are these computers or some other electronic equipment. Whatever they are, the screens are very small', commented Marcelo.

'It looks like they are computers', replied Claire. Early personal computers used to have small screens, small memories and were very slow compared to today's PCs'.

The sign at the entrance door said, on a brand new brass plate: **Forestry Commission**.

At the wide reception desk, there were a middle aged lady and a young one not more than twenty, appearing busy looking at the computer screen while her hands played with the key board.

The older one looked at the four arrivals greeting them with a smile:

'Good morning. How can I help you?'

Carl spoke with the pleasant smile: 'We are interested in to what happened to the clinic that was here many years ago. I suppose you wouldn't know. My friend's wife was treated here about twenty years ago, without success may I say.'

'My colleague here', and she pointed to the young girl typing, 'had not been born yet but I came to work for them just three months before it closed. The Clinic closed in 1987 for refurbishment, we were told but, it never open again. After a while rumors started that it was not up to British medical standards and it was forced to close.'

'Thank you very much. It was very educational', replied Carl.

The four were on their way out when Marcelo excused himself and went back.

'Pardon me but I could not help noticing the brass

plate at the entrance door. It looks almost brand new. Has the Forestry Commission been here long?'

'Oh no sir. We have moved in just six months ago. For a very long time this used to be a Shelter for Battered Wives.'

Marcelo thanked the lady and was ready to rejoin his group when his brain put on the brakes. He turned back and asked:

'The amount of equipment in the skips I noticed is very large. He was searching for a pleasant word to describe the lot but was interrupted:

'No sir, the equipment must have been in the attic for many years. We aim to convert the attic into office space and whatever there was in the attic must have been there since the days of the Clinic, I am sure.'

Marcelo thanked the lady again and rejoined the three waiting beside the car. As Claire and Mathew opened the car door there was a pause, Marcelo appeared as being in a trans.

'Are you all right my friend?', asked Carl.

'Give me a few minutes Carl, I need to use my mobile.'

Marcelo was on the phone for a few minutes while the car occupants waited patiently.

Finally when Marcelo finished phoning, he opened

the car door and said he needed to go back into the building.

About five minutes later when he came out his facial expression changed.

'Carl, could you help me take a few pieces of the electronics from the skip, please, I'll explain later. I asked if I could take some and was told to take anything I wanted.'

Mathew did not have a clue what the old inspector was doing, Carl thought Marcelo might be a collector of junk while Claire kept staring at what Marcelo selected to take.

She came out of the car and coming close to Marcelo asked:

'Do you think it might have belonged to the Clinic inspector?'

'I don't want to raise any hopes but, this opportunity could not be ignored. I see you noticed it as well.'

'I did but, only now. You must have had a suspicion as soon as we arrived here.'

Leaving the car park, Carl asked Marcelo:

'I couldn't help overhearing the name of Gianni when you were phoning. Is he the young computer expert I met at your house Marcelo?'

'He is the one. I asked him if there could be any information stored in the discarded hardware and he said it could be, as people did not pay much attention to clear the hard discs in those days.'

Hearing that, silence grabbed all with each one immersed in their separate thoughts.

Mathew wondered whether all old men collect old bits and pieces and why. Claire prayed that Marcelo finds a way to help get medicine that could help Mathew. Carl was ignorant of any technology but knowing Marcelo, respected and praised his friend's quick thinking and taking the initiative when he noticed the old equipment.

'I think this is all we were able to do today', said Marcelo to break the silence in the car.

My friend, young Gianni will need a day to see if there was anything left on the hard discs and, of course, if it could be retrieved. I will arrange for him to come to London where I'll be staying for a few days. But I will need transport for this "junk" to be brought to London. Could you help me with that Carl?''

'I will bring everything to you tomorrow Marcelo as I will be going back home. But I'll call you to make sure you are at your friends when I come. Is that all right with you?'

'Yes that will be fine Carl.'

The car stopped at Birmingham bus terminal and Marcelo had enough time to smoke a cigarette before boarding the coach for London.

Arriving back to his friends house, Marcelo had to satisfy their curiosity as to why he had to travel to Birmingham and had he found anything. He had to reveal some details because of his need to bring in discarded parts of the old computers he collected from the skip as well.

When Marcelo explained that his colleague Gianni will probably be coming but will stay in a hotel, he was told Gianni could stay with them as it was going to be for a night or two only and there was another spare room in the house.

By the time Carl phoned, Marcelo's mind was in the middle of a fight between the hope that there might be information stored and that it could be retrieved and the dark side, that of fear in finding nothing relevant to the case of the three brothers and the experiments carried during In Vitro Fertilization, if that is what had happened.

Not to be seen in such a mood, Marcelo said to his hosts he was going for a long walk in order to clear his head. He had about half an hour before Carl comes and, not to make Carl wait, he walked up and down the avenue. It was Carl who spotted him and beeped his car horn.

Phoning Gianni and making sure of his coming was another difficult task he had to perform as during the summer months young people like to stay on the beach soaking the sun and doing nothing at all while on their holidays.

But Gianni did respond positively and obtained a cheap weekend return flight from the Ronghi airport near Trieste to Stanstead airport where Marcelo met him.

During the half hour train journey to Liverpool Street Station in London, Marcelo explained the task he hoped Gianni could undertake and possibly obtain some data that could be helpful.

'Will you need anything like tools or equipment. Tony, the friend I am staying with and you will be staying there as well, has set up a PC and a Mac, whatever that means, because he was not sure if the hardware you will work on is suitable for a PC or for Mac. I told Tony I did not know what that meant but he assured me you do.'

'A few cables maybe but, they are not difficult to obtain. Any computer shop would have them', replied Gianni.

Marcelo thought he could start the very next morning but Gianni surprised him by suggesting to look at the equipment within a couple of hours of his arrival to the house.

Seeing the boxes, Gianni told Marcelo he needed some time to try and rig the equipment together and there was no need for the both of them to be there.

Marcelo went to the front room and chatted with

his friend while watching the evening news for about an hour when Gianni came in and said he was ready to proceed with checking the hard discs.

Making the access to the hard disc of the first piece of the equipment it indicated there was material stored. Gianni was able, without effort, to bring a sample to the screen and it looked like a short letter but unfortunately it was coded.

It wasn't a code with, say, a fixed number of symbols in each group but, just like a text, some "words" were short and some long just like an ordinary written text but instead of letters only, the text contained numbers and letters in every word

There was a word written on top right hand corner of the screen GERMANICUS

'Gianni, I have a feeling I saw something like this before.'

Suddenly it came to him.

Way back when he was a young school boy in the fifth grade, Marcelo, like other boys and girls of that age, started sending short notes to each other in the class for the first time.

It became a fashion to do so at that age and the couple would make up a code in which they would write to each other notes. The text was innocent in itself but, the code made it exciting and mysterious.

For example a code using letters in a word GERMANICUS would be matched with numbers 9 to 0 and every time that a letter came up in a word to be one from the word the code represented, it was replaced by the equivalent number.

So a note: you are beautiful would be written as: y09 532 b259t7f9l.

Looking at the screen, everything was coded except the names of three people that might have been medics.

Two of the names appeared to be of Italian origin and Marcelo closed his eyes and tried to recall as many ten letter codes as he could from his childhood. Every time one came up he wrote it down and so on until his mind was exhausted and he went out to have a cigarette.

Coming back in and staring at the new text on the screen, Marcelo noticed, at the top right hand corner what appeared to be a title of some sort.

Seven Christmases

To start with it did not mean anything but, slowly Marcelo realized it could be the code.

Looking at the code words from his childhood, there was a code CETIMANOLS. In the jargon terms it should have meant *cetima* meaning seven and *nols* as noels

There was a coded text covering about half of a page and Marcelo tried to decode it using the above code word.

The signature was written as 541h629. Using the code it read: Michael.

With the excitement Marcelo lit a cigarette and then realized he shouldn't have while in the house.

Gianni was out and it appeared ages to Marcelo. On his return, Marcelo took him to the computer and asked:

'Gianni, could it be possible to use the code here for you to change the coded text into a normal one?'

'I'll try but, I need to do a few things first. Give me half an hour and I'll give you an answer.'

It took Gianni a few hours to write a program and when he was finished, he called Marcelo and sitting down in front of the screen, highlighted a page Marcelo pointed out and then pressed a few keys, saying he was now changing the language of the text into plain English.

Suddenly there it was, a new page of normal readable text:

Tim

The last experiment did not work. The fertilized egg survived only a day.

We have to reduce the dosage strength by, say, ten times and if there are multiple

divisions and the egg survives for at least four days we
may change the parameters again then.

If there is no improvement, reduce the dosage strength by
another ten times.

Make sure you keep accurate records.

Surrounding temperature must be 37 degrees centigrade
within the limits we set.

Will have another meeting on Friday.
Michael

'Gianni you are a genius. Is that all I need to do with
the rest?'

'If the code is the same for all the text here then that
is all you need to do but, maybe it would be better if I do
it for you as you might erase the original text and then
there would be nothing to decode.'

'You don't think much of my computer knowledge,
do you Gianni. Fair enough, let us leave it for tomorrow
and I will wait for you to finish. After that you may go
sight seeing or anything you like. Is that all right with
you?'

Next morning Gianni was up early and by the time
Marcelo had his breakfast the whole coded text had been
decoded and ready for Marcelo to engage with.

Gianni took the second hard disc out from the box of
four Marcelo rescued from the skip, but here the solution

required a different approach and different decoding formula.

'Marcelo, I think the best thing would be if you put effort into finding the code word for each of the hard discs and I will then convert the coded text into plain English. Then my work will be finished and you can continue in peace.'

'Yes I'll do that. You go and enjoy yourself but be back after lunch when I might hopefully have something for you to do.'

But this time it was much harder to find the key to decode the text.

What looked like a hint for the medics all those years ago, was a sign on the top right hand corner of the screen saying: "**Forest sirens**".

Marcelo tried all he could but nothing matched, not even close.

He was in two minds whether to consult with Gianni to take the hard discs with him and try to extract the data back home when his mobile phone rang. It was Carl calling from France enquiring if there has been any progress.

'Initially we got one of the hard discs sorted out and there is quite a bit to study but, now we, or better, I am stuck and don't know where to go from here. But give me time and I hope I'll have something for you.'

'Listen Marcelo. Why don't you bring Gianni here and he can spend a few days on the beach as well as helping you?'

'I have to think about it Carl. Gianni came here for a weekend only and wouldn't be fair to force him. I'll let you know in a day or so.'

'Marcelo', said Gianni, could the sirens refer to girls. You know the Greek stories about the mermaids? I have never heard of forest mermaids but you could try anyhow while I sort out your first and second hard disc and print what is there.'

Marcelo looked at the screen for about two hours when he heard Gianni's suggestion. He was going to reject it when a tune came to his head of a very popular song. Popular, that is, about fifty years ago: La Boscaiola.

He wrote it down and noticed there was the letter "a" repeated three times. There were eleven letters as well. He was going to discard it and then he saw it.

L'Boscarine is the same meaning but is spelled in the northern dialect in Italy and, of course, forest sirens is plural so the last letter of the code word should be a letter e. He tried a few coded words and 'bingo'.

'Gianni you were right. At least it works for this page. Could you, when you can, try if it is the same for the whole disc please, I need a cigarette without delay?'

And Marcelo went out to the garden.

Gianni used the same program for decoding as he did the previous day except the ten symbols which he, this time, replaced with the word "lboscarine".

The whole disc was tested just by looking at the text and everything was legible although the text was full of errors.

But Marcelo was quick to notice that in order to make it more difficult to be deciphered, the medics used their knowledge of Italian language spoken in the north and distorted the English words, in a similar way as the Italian people pronounce them.

Gianni connected the fourth disc and there was the same note at the top right hand corner of the screen: Forest sirens.

Within a minute the text was decoded and, the same with the fourth disc.

Gianni stored the text from each hard disc onto a memory stick and marked the source.

'Marcelo here is everything that was on the hard discs you found. You may throw the old staff away or keep it. You never know if Carl might need or want the originals.'

It was Saturday night and Marcelo and Gianni were invited by their host for a drink in the local pub.

Both of them were delighted with the atmosphere in the pub but did not enjoy their drinks.

When asked do they normally have beer, Marcelo explained that beer, back home, is usually drank in the summer and for that reason it is always drank cold. Not to show any disrespect, Marcelo added:

'Both Gianni and myself are not the right ones to compare the drinks here with the ones at home as we both prefer wine and only when having dinner.'

Next morning Gianni left to take the train to Stanstead airport and Marcelo was to travel by train to La Rochele where Carl was to meet him and take him back to his house.

The equipment Marcelo posted was to take a few days to arrive but the two friends were looking forward to study the text obtained from the old, discarded computers of almost twenty years back.

Marcelo went out into the garden to have a cigarette and sitting down on a wooden bench that Carl made himself, drifted into the past when he was promoted and took over his first case of burglary with homicide.

The shotgun that was used in the murder was found near the body and somebody's fingerprints were still on the trigger. There was a suspect, a young man by the name of Trost. He was brought in and fingerprinted but they did not match the ones on the gun. Marcelo could not sleep for days as, his instincts were telling him the main suspect was the murderer and the investigation traveled in an ever increased circles without any progress.

Finally he decided to check every step taken since the beginning of the investigation and on Marcelo's insistence, the men involved presented every detail of their work.

The technician that took fingerprints of the suspects was a young graduate who proudly stated he remembered all the details, especially that of taking the fingerprints of the then main suspect because the man spilled the ink and his fingers got saturated with the liquid and had to wipe the excess of the ink from his fingers with a cloth.

Everything was suddenly clear. Marcelo told two of his colleagues to go and arrest the man Trost who was main suspect to start with. When he was brought in, first he complained of harassment as he was already cleared and then refused to be fingerprinted again saying he had already volunteered and that it had been done when he was brought to the police station last time. To his demand for his layer, Marcelo said:

Of course Mr Trost. Here is the phone and you call your layer.'

On the arrival of the layer, Marcelo took out of his pocket a strip of developed film with a few negatives on it.

'You see young man', started Marcelo. ' this is proof

that you pulled that trigger and killed the innocent man.'

The young Trost laughed and advised his solicitor sitting beside him to lodge a complaint of harassment but Marcelo continued.

'This black and white negative is called negative because it reverses the effect of light exposing the areas of the film. The image here depicts a person who has dark hair. On the negative here it looks as if the hair is grey. The person is Caucasian and yet the negative presents his face as black. That is because the negative reverses the light of the image photographed.

You young man were fingerprinted but you cleverly created a negative image of your fingerprints. You have done this by saturating your fingers with excess of ink and then wiping the excess ink off your fingers. This way your fingers had the ink in the grooves of your finger's skin and not on top.

Your solicitor here should advice you that your fingerprints could be taken by force if you don't want to do it willingly.'

'My I have a few minutes with my client inspector?', asked the solicitor, and Marcelo and his colleague left the room.

Coming back in after five minutes, Marcelo was told by the solicitor that his client wants to plead guilty to manslaughter which was done in self defense when the murdered man ran towards his client with a knife.

'Your client will be charged with murder. He has killed an innocent man who was an invalid and who was not able to even get up from his chair without help', and Marcelo switched the recording apparatus off and called two officers to take the accused to the police cell.

The young police officer that made a blunder with the original fingerprinting came to Marcelo with the intention of apologizing but Marcelo stopped him saying:

'We all learn from our mistakes. This might be your first one but it is definitely not the last. The main think is to learn from them and not to repeat them.'

'Are you talking to yourself Marcelo?', asked Carl hearing the last sentence Marcelo uttered without realizing his thoughts were actually audible.

'Carl, my friend, what I find difficult to take is when somebody does a bad thing to another human being knowing very well that what he or she is doing is evil. That is when my adrenaline level raises and I could not stop until I find the culprit.'

Irene, Ann and Amanda have agreed and made an appointment for the three boys to be examined in the London clinic where Joe had his tests. But in order for the three to have the tests the same day, there was a date set and they had to wait until the end of the month, seventeen long days.

The mothers had copies of all the medical histories of their boys ready and, a day before the appointment at the London clinic, met at the hotel situated at the walking distance from the clinic not far from the famous Oxford Street.

One word could describe the feeling of the three mothers:

Fear!

Each one was scared and fearful of the unknown and of hearing the results of the tests.

Irene had her grandmother in a home and used to visit her there regularly. The old people used to sit in the large room or hall, TV set was on but there was no normal conversation. Some people would talk to themselves, some would talk as if there are others listening but majority would just sit and stare, nowhere in particular, or dozing until they were moved either back to their rooms or to the dining hall.

Looking at the three boys, Irene could not help but to draw similarities and that scared her even more.

Neither of the mothers slept much and needed some time to sort their faces in the morning.

Coming to the clinic, the receptionist was ready for them and the mothers were invited to come for a chat with the consultants Mr Atkinson and Mr Thorn.

'Ladies, my colleague Mr Atkinson and myself wanted to give you a timetable of the tests which will last for three days about three hours each day, with most tests being carried out in the mornings.

First of all we will take a sample of the boys DNAs and by the end of the tests we will have some results from their DNA analysis. We understand you were told that the boys metabolisms are ageing faster than normal. We hope that the DNA tests will be able to give us a more detailed picture as well as other tests like the CT scan, blood analysis and many other tests applied during the next three days. If any of you have any queries or questions this might be appropriate time to ask.'

Irene was the bravest after a period of silence and she asked if it was possible for a boy of such a young age to be prone to any brain waste disease.

'My boy's mental power in remembering music has been exceptional', and here she paused. 'but the last year or so it became harder and harder for him to do that.'

'No Mrs Taylor. Normally the brain is still not at its peak at the age of twenty. But if there are symptoms, something else could be the cause and we hope the tests will reveal as to what could cause this effect.'

'I read about premature ageing and then there was a program on the television that scared me to death. But the children there looked different.'

'You are probably talking about the disease called Progeria, Mrs Brown.

Progeria is a disease that affects about one in four million people and there are only forty or so known cases in the world and the average life expectancy for someone with this condition is about thirteen to fourteen years of age.

The disease does not show at birth but soon, i.e. within the first year, the face expression changes and baldness appears with aged looking skin, dwarfism and a small face and jaw relative to head size. It never comes in more than one child in a family although, may I add, that there is a case in Asia where a number of siblings appear to have Progeria but, it is actually a fault in the DNA structure, different to Progeria.'

'How could a young child age fast?', asked Amanda with a frightened voice.

'As we grow up, the cells in our body divide so that new ones could replace the worn out or damaged ones but, this could only be achieved a predefined number of times. As we age, cells lose the ability to multiply or, should I say divide.

If there is a fault in a particular place in our DNA structure, the cells could divide much faster and thus die faster as well. It is this process which might lead to premature ageing.'

'Is it inherited, I mean passed down from the parents?', asked Irene.

'No Mrs Brown. It is caused by a random genetic defect. Your son inherited almost half of his genes from you and half from his father. I say almost because some of his genes have mutated and that gives him his unique DNA chart. The mutated genes do, although very seldom, go wrong, if I may use the term, and the result shows sometime during the life of the person.'

The silence was so powerful that the consultants, having experienced similar situations many a time, changed the subject and invited the three mothers to see the medical instruments their children will be tested with knowing perfectly well that this calms patients as well as their families.

Carol Paterson was determined to find out why were so many mistakes made in the case of the three babies and their mother and the adopting parents.

Not one but three times was the death of Sharon written into birth certificates of the three babies and yet there was no evidence of Sharon's death certificate in any of the three documents.

Carol searched the files in the Register of Births in Hereditch but was told they must have been transferred as the data were removed from the file.

In the Children Society there was a note but written by one of the then staff members.

The Children Society has been informed that the mother of the babies Mathew, Tom and Joe now placed for adoption had died giving birth.

There were no details as to where the information came from and no documents were in the file.

Never in her sixteen years experience as counselor had she come across a case where so many documents have disappeared and she was determined to ensure that the authorities tighten the rules so that it could never happen again.

She even visited the boys' mother, Sharon. She appeared as clear minded as a normal person chatting to a nurse.

After enquiring about the nurse Ruth, Carol was told the nurse in question has not been on duty for three weeks now without any notice and her employment had been terminated.

Carol got attached to Mathew and felt she let him down although there was nothing more she could do.

Mathew, in her opinion, was very clever but sensitive and probably vulnerable.

He, Carol thought, was lucky to have found a girl like Claire.

She wrote a long letter explaining the dead ends she

encountered in her search but at the end decided to invite Mathew to her office and pass the information, or the lack of it, to him orally first. Three days in a row she tried his home the number but there was no answer.

Her summer holidays were approaching and as it was almost a year since she was at Mathew's and Claire's wedding she went out and found a beautiful wedding anniversary card which she addressed to Mathew and Claire saying she will give them a call on her return from holidays.

Carl and Marcelo had been reading the printouts Gianni obtained from the old computers Marcelo managed to rescue from the skip, but the contents did not make much sense to either of them.

There were many words which sounded like sophisticated chemical compound and Marcelo suggested to halt the reading and think of an alternative.

'What do you have in mind my friend?', asked Carl.

'Well, if we could find a trusted chemist or biochemist, I think we might get much more out of all this instead of us prodding in the dark.'

'There is a chemist here on the peninsula. He had retired about four years ago and I meet him occasionally when we play for a monthly medal at the golf course where we are both members. I'll see if he would be willing to help us.'

'Dinner is served, gentlemen!', announced Tania just as the two men were going through the back door into the garden.

'Tania and Ida are so close as if they knew each other for ever', said Carl.

'Yes they are but, I think we should look into a flight back. I feel Tania is missing our grandchildren and probably her own house as well.'

Sitting at the dining table, Carl had to get up again as the phone, on the hall stand, rang.

He wasn't there for more than a couple of minutes and coming back to the table said:

'We are having visitors tonight. Francois and Gilbert are coming for a drink after eight.'

Tania was ready to suggest to Marcelo for the two of them to go for a walk when Carl added that Gilbert was the chemist he was talking about to Marcelo.

'I explained to him about the contents of the material Marcelo obtained and how we could not make heads or tails out of it and he offered to have a look.'

As it was only early afternoon, the Campbells invited Marcelo and Tania sightseeing along the peninsula coast. Of course they had to drive as the journey would have taken them far too long if they walked.

'Everything here reminds us of our visit to Croatia except the sea', stated Ida.

'Here the sea is always rough while your Adriatic sea is so calm one can imagine that it might be possible to walk on it.'

'Well, you should see it in the winter when the north wind called "bura" blows', responded Tania and everybody laughed.

Soon it was time to turn back and receive Francois and Gilbert.

After the introductions, they sat in the garden with a glass of desert wine and engaged in small talk. Everything was lovely except that Marcelo's and Tania's French was poor and Francois and Gilbert were about the same trying using English.

But when it came to reading, Gilbert had no problem which he explained was due to doing a lot of studying from English books.

'This is incorrect English, no', was Gilbert's comment after coming to a word that the original writers used.

After going through a dozen pages of, mostly short notes or letters, Gilbert announced that it looks as if there were experiments being carried out on either rabbits or some other animals.

'Ui mon ami. There is only one thing strange. Whoever wrote this, must have been a lover of animals as he used human names and sometimes even surnames to point out which animal had been used.'

Carl and Marcelo looked at each other and Carl said:

'Gilbert, this work had been carried out in a clinic involved in InVitro Fertilization.'

'No, no my friend. It is not allowed to expose either the egg or sperm used for the IVF to chemicals, especially the ones mentioned here and in such dozes. No, I do not believe it.'

'What if I tell you that it was done almost twenty years ago?'

Gilbert closed his eyes for a moment and then said:

'Twenty years ago there was talk about the possibility of creating a, how do you say in English, "made to order babies". But to do what says here was and still is a criminal act and any medic doing it would be, at least, expelled from the medical profession.

I am speaking for the medical ethics here in France but I am sure they are the same in England.'

'Gilbert, could you look at the written material we have here and make a summary of what you think was going on in the clinic, please? There are about one hundred twenty pages in all.'

'Of course my friend. It will take me about a week

or so because, as you know, my wife and I are in the competition in our golf club.'

'Whenever you can, it will be fine with me Gilbert.'

Carl printed all the material he and Marcelo retrieved from the discarded parts of the clinic's computers and gave it to Gilbert before the visitors departed.

Marcelo asked Carl if he could look at the flights on the internet and obtaining the tickets, he and Tania departed on the afternoon the following day.

'Carl I would like to know what happens with all this. Could you keep me informed please?'

'Of course I will. And I hope we will be fishing from your boat next summer when Francois and I come, as promised.'

It was the third and final day of the tests and the three mothers were dreading the afternoon meeting with the consultants.

While the boys were being tested and the results ana-lysed, the mothers went to a nearby café to console each other and gather strength.

At one in the afternoon they collected the boys from the clinic and took them to a quiet little restaurant for lunch.

Looking at the menu in front of them, the boys did not show any interest in choosing themselves. When Ann suggested to Joe to have a steak and chips, suddenly the problem was solved as the other boys said they were going to have the same.

It was sad for the mothers to see their sons without the vigour young boys normally have and it was a blessing that they agreed to come to the clinic together. This way it was a little easier to carry the burden of fear of their boys uncertain future.

When rested, the boys still looked their own age except for Joe who, in the last eighteen months, sagged from his physical strength of an eighteen year old athlete to a worn out late thirties man.

Amanda's face could not hide her fear and worry. She loved her Mathew even more now than when he was a small boy of six showing, already then, his possible potential in numerical skills. And she was worried for Claire, her daughter in law who fulfilled Mathew's life.

'Are you all right Mathew?', whispered Amanda seeing her son immersed in thoughts.

'Yes mum but, I miss Claire. She is working today so I'll phone her after six when she will be back at our apartment.'

'Not to worry. We will have a nice rest tonight and then the journey home will not be so tiresome.'

'What were they looking for by doing all those tests

on us?', asked Tom and, it was a thought his two brothers wanted to ask as well.

Irene was the quickest to find the way out.

'You Tom, and your two brothers as well, started to get tired very easily lately and we thought it might help the doctors if they see all of you together.'

'Did you tell them that our doctor mentioned the possibility I might have glandular fever?'

'Yes I did and they were going to look if that might have been the case with you.'

'What is glandular fever, mum?', asked Joe.

Ann looked at Irene and then back at her son when Irene spoke.

'It is something that stays inside you after you have a cold and makes you feel tired.

That is all Joe.'

Ann looked at Irene and gave her a thankful nod.

'Look how time flies' exclaimed Irene after checking her wrist watch. 'We have to get back to the clinic.'

After paying for the food and drinks, the three boys with their mothers put on their coats and walked back towards the clinic each boy holding his mother's hand.

On their arrival to the clinic, the boys were given a room with many journals connected with sports, films, art and many other subjects.

'We will take your mothers and have a chat with

them for about half an hour', explained Mr Thorn, 'you entertain yourselves and if you need anything, ask our beautiful Marion. She will look after you'

'Come in ladies, please.'

As the mothers sat down, and the consultants took their seats behind a wide desk, the silence starting to hurt.

Mr Thorn's experience made him expect anxiety felt by the three ladies but the intensity surprised even him. But he took control and addressed the mothers.

'Ladies, first let me say that this was the most comprehensive set of tests my colleague and I undertook.

This we did because here we have three young boys with similar and yet different symptoms of being unwell and the effects of these symptoms are different to each boy.

Because the boys lived all their lives separate from one another, we studied the areas for any known data on chemical pollution but could not trace any.

The tests on any irregular patterns show the boys skin, bones, outside and inside organs have no known diseases or any irregular structures.'

This statement made the mothers breathe again. Up to now they were like statuettes made from ice.

But that soon changed as the consultant continued.

'There was only one thing out of place the DNA charts

showed and even that would have been impossible to find if we didn't look for the symptoms of premature ageing what was suggested by the Chester clinic colleagues.

The defect in the DNA structure causing premature ageing has been discovered very recently and when we looked for it, neither of the three boys have any defects at that point in their DNA structure.

This is what we found this is what my colleague and I will try to explain to you.

In the chain of the DNA where the defect causes premature ageing, there are about a thousand links and only two, that is if known to be defected using up to date medical knowledge, cause premature ageing or **Progeria.** I may safely say that your boys have no defects there.

Now, this is where the problem starts. There are a few defects a bit farther away from the one causing Progeria in all your boys but, what is so strange, each boy has the defects at different parts of the DNA chain.

We can with definitive assurance state that it could not have been inherited. We already said that environment did not cause that, so the last option, Mr Atkinson and myself believe might be that your boys were conceived by IVF treatment and that there was chemistry influencing the defects in the structure I mentioned. Different chemicals could have interfered with egg or sperm or even later after the egg had been fertilized. This could have been done either by accident or we fear it could have been done on purpose.

Do you have any knowledge of how did their mother conceive?'

After a long pause, Irene managed to get enough breath to say.

'Each one of us were told the boy's mother died at birth and nobody mentioned the triplets and.'

'My son found out he was adopted and started to question the Child Registry and after their eighteenth birthday it became known that their mother was still alive and that there were two more brothers.'

Maybe my son Mathew could tell us if there are any data on that.' uttered Amanda in a low frightened voice.

'Could you ask your son to come in please Mrs Williams?', asked Mr Atkinson.

'Young man', asked Mr Thorn when Mathew sat down beside his mother.

'Do you know how your mother, I mean your birth mother', the consultant corrected himself, seeing a strange look on Mathew's face, 'how did she become pregnant?'

'She couldn't, not for many years. Then a clinic offered her and her husband money and made it possible.'

'You mean she had to pay for the treatment, don't you?'

'No, they helped her get pregnant for free and they

paid her money as well saying something like she would be a special case or something like that. I think that is what happened but Carl Campbell would know more. I am not sure anymore.'

'And who is Mr Campbell, Mathew?'

'Oh, he was a friend of my …and he looked at Amanda…of my birth father and birth mother and he was their solicitor.' Looking at Amanda he added.

'Claire could tell you more. I think she even writes to Mr Campbell.'

That is fine Mathew. Your mother will ask Claire to send me Mr Campbell's address and we will proceed from there. You can go and join your brothers and your mother will be out shortly.'

The two consultants exchanged a few looks and then Mr Thorn addressed the mothers again.

'Dear ladies, this is a very special case even for us as we have never encountered anything similar. My colleague Mr Atkinson and myself would like very much to do a thorough study of the boys case and are prepared to offer it to you free of charge.

Would you like us to undertake this work for you. It might not bring any help in treating your boys but, at least, you might be able to know the reasons for your boys condition.'

The three mothers did not expect anything like this

and after exchanging a few glances accepted the consultant's offer wholeheartedly.

'Mr Thorn, I will get the address of Mr Campbell from my daughter in law and send it to you. I think that Mr Campbell has done something already and has involved a detective as well, who is a friend of his. I hope he will be able to give you additional answers himself.'

The three mothers left the consulting room, collected their boys and traveled separately to their homes.

Mr Thorn looked at his colleague, Mr Atkinson, when the mothers departed and, who commented:

'Henry, we will have to thread very carefully as it might come out as, potentially, a very hot subject.'

'I was thinking along the same line. Before we publish anything, we must be very sure of the data obtained.'

Carl Campbell was trying to decide what to do with the written material Marcelo was able to retrieve from the rescued twenty years old computers discarded outside the Clinic's former building as he, himself, could not be either moral or ethical judge of the work described in the written data.

He felt bad even about thinking of sending the written material to Mathew when Claire, phoned.

She described the visit by the three brothers to the London clinic and the probable diagnosis of their condition and future prospects. When she suggested to send any data that were gotten from the junk computers to the London Clinic, Carl was delighted to tell her there was quite a lot rescued by the detective and was to send everything to the consultants she mentioned.

But to his surprise, he received a letter from London in an official envelope he recognized as that of the clinic Claire mentioned.

Running their own clinic made the two consultants work long hours and neither had published a single scientific paper for over three years since the clinic was established.

This was one of the reasons for their interest in the case of the three boys although, they honestly felt that the case should be investigated and published if there were unethical methods used by the clinic where the three boys were conceived using IVF method.

When the data, retrieved from the discarded computers and posted by Carl Campbell, arrived the two consultants spent a late evening scanning through.

But soon decided they needed more time and cancelled their last daily consulting appointments in order to dedicate more time to the analysis of the work carried out twenty years previously.

'This was not an IVF Clinic, Henry. This was a laboratory with guinea pigs substituted by embryos, fertilized eggs, foetuses and even unborn babies with their mothers being up to twelve weeks pregnant. This wasn't medical research either, according to these notes. It was like a dentist learning how to extract a tooth through you know what. My God Adam, I wish we could find out who did this and expose them.'

'Listen Ian, we are not that busy in the next couple of days. What about you taking the few patients I have in my diary and I try to find out who ran the clinic and where are they now?

'Done! But no more than two days as I promised my family a trip to France and I could not get out of it this time.'

The very first thing Henry Thorn did was to find the list of Clinics dating twenty years back.

It took him best part of the first day to locate a Clinic First English American Medical Services (FEAMS).

The Clinic was located in Hereditch, just south of Birmingham.

The Clinic was active for about seven years but nothing else was known besides its name and IVF as its field of medical research.

Mr Thorn tried to find out if there were any names of patients or clients but that information was not available either. There was just a list of four directors, with addresses, one in the United States, two in Italy and two in England.

The one in the USA could not, after twenty years, be traced, two addresses in Italy did not and, apparently, never existed and one director in England died nine years ago without a family.

At the very last address given, there still lived at present his wife, looked after by her daughter.

The two medics traveled to Fleetwood, a small town which twenty years previously used to be a small fishing village, but that industry disappeared with the lack of fishing stock.

When Messrs Atkinson and Thorn called at the house and presented their business cards, the daughter thought they were, after they introduced themselves, to see her mother.

'Mrs Richards, my colleague Mr Atkinson and myself are trying to find as much as possible about the early IVF treatment as we are writing a book on the history of IVF. Could you tell us what you remember from the years when your husband was one of the directors at the Hereditch Clinic please?

'It was a very modern but small Clinic as far as I could remember but, that is about all. My husband did not want to bring his work home, as he used to say', replied Mrs Richards in her slow speech.

'What about the babies? Were there any twins born as it became a case with later clinical IVF treatments?

'There were no babies born! My dad told me, once when I asked him that, the clinic was doing studies or something like that but not making babies for people who could not have them normally.' said Helen, the daughter.

As they were leaving the daughter asked:

Will the book be out soon? My mother would like to see our dad's name in print. He has been dead for eleven years already and we both miss him very much.

'We are sorry to hear that. When the book is out we will send you a copy. Thank you very much for seeing us.

On their way back to London, the two consultants debated the meeting and concluding that if they were to continue search, a lot more time was needed to be spent what they could not afford.

When Helen brought her mother the afternoon tea, Mrs Richards said:

'They did not ask about dad's colleagues! They could have probably told them much more as your dad was involved in the Clinic for the first three years only.'

'Maybe they were in touch with uncle Michael and uncle Lauro already.'

'It would be nice to see them again Helen. Wouldn't it. They always talk nice about your dad.'

A week later just when Helen brought her mother her breakfast upstairs, the phone rang and she rushed downstairs to the hall to answer it.

'Hello! Said Helen lifting the phone.

'Happy birthday young girl! Said a male voice and Helen immediately recognized it.

'Hello uncle Lauro. Thank you very much. You remem-ber my birthday every year. You have never for-gotten it all these years.'

'I have it imprinted in my mind and it reminds me every year. And how is your mum?'

'She is fine really fine. Oh I almost forgot. There will be a book. Two men are writing it and you will be in it.'

'Oh! How do you know?'

'Well they came here. I mean the two men that are writing the book. They said something about the history of IVF or something like that. They talked to mum and me and promised us they will send us a copy when it is published.'

'Did they say who they were. I mean their names?'

'No they didn't but they left their business cards. They came from London.'

....

'Uncle Lauro, are you still there?

274

'Yes I am sweetheart. Listen, send me the details from their cards and I will get in touch with them to see if they would like any more information for their book.'

'Silly me! I should have thought of it and given them your name. I am sorry I completely forgot.

Helen copied the men's cards onto her computer and sent an email to her "uncle Lauro" thanking him for remembering her birthday.

Henry Taylor did not mention to his colleague that he managed to get the addresses of the two directors of the FEAMS, those with nonexisting addresses in Italy. He succeeded to trace them to the Costa dell Sol in Spain.

Something else Mr Taylor did not mention to his colleague as well.

Henry Taylor was a gambler. Not one of those playing slot machines, no horseracing betting and no poker or any other card games. In fact he gambled on his own in his home, using internet. It had been going on for a few years by now.

He owed large sums of money to a number of banks and some of the banks were ready to take him to court to force him to pay their money back.

When he heard about the Clinic in Hereditch and its history, Henry Thorp developed a plan in his mind within two days and saw his future sorted out. He was able to get the mobile phone number of Michael Gardena, one of the directors in the Clinic.

He started realizing his plan.

'Dr Gardena?

'Yes, who is it?

The subject is FEAMS. Do you want to talk about it or shall I go to the press?

'I don't know what you are talking about, but go on!

'That's better! I am coming to see you and you prepare fifty thousand euro. In return I will give you all the documents and the correspondence recovered from the computers you left when your "Clinic" closed. Your coding was very primitive.'

There was a pause and then the voice said:

'OK but, how will I know that what you bring will be all you have in your possesion?

'Because I say so"

'OK, when could you come?

'When will you have the money?

'Come on Thursday. Give me a call when you arrive!

'Thursday it is then!

Henry went home, got his flight ticket to Malaga for the following Thursday, booked a car at Malaga airport for two days and dreamt about his coming fortune.

By coincidence, his partner left with his family, to

drive to the south of France where they had their summer house.

Arriving to Malaga airport, he collected his car and then phoned Dr Gardena and was given the name of the place where they were to meet.

Driving on the right was a new experience for him and seeing a respectable man holding his thumb up at the side of the A366 road towards a place called Coin, he stopped and the hitchhiker smiled and asked for a lift to Ojen.

Henry was pleased hearing american accent which meant he could have a conversation while traveling to meet his "donor"

'What are you doing here in Spain? Asked the hitch hiker after Henry Thorp told him he had just arrived from London.

'I am living my chilhood for a few days. I used to hitch hike through Europe when I finished my college and spent couple of days here around Costa del Sol.' 'Here; would like special chocolate?

And the hitch hiker took out of his shoulder bag a nice looking box full of different chocolate shapes. Taking one, he offered the box to Henry.

Taking one, Henry had to agree they tasted super.

'May I bother you by asking you to pull at the sign where it says toilette, my bladder is playing on me lately.

Henry felt a bit dizzy and it suited him to have a short break as well and pulled into a layby and his guest went to the loo.

Henry opened the car window and put his head back and closed his eyes. Within a minute he was gone.

The "american" checked there were no cars coming, pulled Henry's body out of the car, dragged it into the bushes and drove away.

Later on in the evening the citizens of the town of Coin noticed fire in the field and youngsters ran towards it and noticed it was a car. As the number plates were removed, it took four days for the car to be identified as the one rented from the Malaga airport.

Monday morning Ian Atkinson was late coming to the Clinic but was surprised seeing people gathering outside and two police cars parked in front of the entrance.

When he was, on his arrival, asked by the police to move on, he replied he was the owner of the Clinic. Mr Atkinson was then shown where to park and was escorted into the premises.

There was a total chaos in the Clinic.

All filling cabinets empty and paperwork scattered across the floor. Medical instruments were on the floor, some turned over but, to the surprise of the police and Mr Atkinson, nothing was broken or damaged.

'Mr Atkinson, could you tell us whether you think anything is missing?

But Mr Atkinson could not speak. He was dumb-founded. He could not understand why would somebody do this. It appeared as a prank with nothing broken but everything displaced giving appearance of hate towards the Clinic.

'I have no idea why anybody would do such a thing" uttered Mr Atkinson. 'Maybe my partner would know. I'll try and get him on the phone.'

After a while he went to the police officer and said:

'I can't understand. My partner, Mr Thorp, should have been here before me and I tried his home and his mobile phone but there is no answer.

When Mr Thorp did not appear by twelve o'clock, the police asked for his address and went to investigate. To their surprise there was no answer and, trying to find out why the break in at the Clinic occurred, they forced the door in.

The appartment was empty as if nobody lived there for some time. The small office on the other hand was very untidy compared to the rest of the appartment.

There was nothing the police could find but fix the door to be locked again, place a notice on the door for Mr Thorp to contact the police and they drove back to the Clinic.

'Mr Atkinson, how well do you know Mr Thorp?

'Well we are sharing this Clinic, being equal partners but, because Mr Thorp has no family he has separate circle of friends. We do meet playing golf occasionally but are not playing in same foursome.

He is a very professional medic if I may say so.'

'Is he a ladies man"

'He has had lady friends but never anyone that I know too serious. Is there something wrong at his appartment?

'We did not find him there.

As there was no trace of Mr Thorp's steps, the police called for the special unit to search his appartment to see if anything could come out of it. At the same time they kept an eye on Mr Atkinson.

It could not be dismissed that Mr Atkinson might be involved in the dissapearance of his partner.

Next day Mrs Atkinson called her husband before he left for work and whispered.

'Ian, there is a car across the road with two people in it. I feel they are observing our house.'

'Well, just in case, ask for identity before opening the door when I am not here.

When he left, his wife noticed that the car, after about less than half a minute followed in the same direction. She took the phone and dialed her husband's mobile.

Ian, the car that was across the road. I think they are following you. What will you do?

'Don't worry! I will stop at the nearest police station.'

Parking in front of the police building he noticed that the car that was following stopped about hundred metres back.

Many police officers do not know what stands for Mr in medical profession so he said coming to the reception desk.

'My name is Dr Atkinson. I am being followed. There is a car parked over there', and he described the car, 'and has followed me from my house all the way here. I would be grateful if you can do something about it.'

Being able to read the registration plate from the office window, police officer lifted the phone and in less than minute was told it was a car used by the police.

Arriving to his Clinic, he noticed another, this time a marked police car just outside the entrance.

An officer cought up with him as Mr Atkinson was going through the door and addressed him.

'Mr Atkinson, we are sorry for you not being told that we placed an unmarked police car outside your house. It was just a precaution, you understand.

'Any news about my colleague Mr Thorp? I still couldn't get in touch with him.'

'We are still looking for him and will let you know if we find him.'

Ian Atkinson felt very uncomfortable feeling that police suspect that he might be connected with his partner's dissapearance especially when the next morning they came to the Clinic again.

'Mr Atkinson did you know that Mr Thorp booked a flight to Spain on the day you told us you departed with your family for your four day break to France?

'No I did not. He was supposed to carry on with his and my patients booked for last Thursday and Friday.'

'Do you know if he has anybody he was going to?

'I am afraid I do not. But why all these questions?

'Well, we found that he booked a car to be collected at Malaga airport. He booked it for two days but the car has not so far been returned.'

'I am in the dark as much as you are inspector.'

'Mr Atkinson, may ask you, did you travel to Spain while on your holidays in the south of France?

'For God's sake inspector! There are at least four people, not counting my family, I spent with during our stay in France. I'll give you a list and you go and talk to them. Anything else?

'No! Not for now Mr Atkinson. Thank you for your time and cooperation.'

Ian Atkinson was raging. Just as the business has

established itself and their reputation attracted many patients, this happened. Why would his partner suddenly leave and not mention anything to him. After all, all business decisions were always with joint agreement and they had no secrets. His partner seemed to be extravagant in spending his own money but he was an honest man.

'Hello! Said Tania breathless as she rushed downstairs and lifted the phone.

'Hello Tania! This is Carl. How are you, and how is Marcelo?

'We are both fine Carl. Are you all packed. We are waiting for you to come.

'We are planing to leave on Monday and hope to be with you on Wednesday. Would that be all right with you and Marcelo?

'Of course Carl! Looking forward to you coming. Give my love to Ida.'

Marcelo was delighted. He liked Carl as a friend and fishing together from the same boat is much more pleasing than being on his own. And going on a few days cruise will be so much more enjoyable. He wrote the items needed to be sorted out on the boat.

The automatic pilot has already been looked at and was in order. The engine had been serviced, battery, the an "accumulator" as Marcelo called it has been installed and a new fridge fitted. Marcelo ordered a new DC/AC converter so that any appliance used at home, could be used on board as well.

Tania made sure the bedding was as it should be and Marcelo prepared all fishing gear, he and Carl were going to use.

Wednesday afternoon, with temperatures soaring to the high thirtees, the French visitors arrived. Marcelo helped Carl with unpacking while Tania took Ida to take her to have a cold drink.

Was the journey hard Ida? Asked Tania.

'Yes and no. It was long but the motorways are now covering almost the whole journey and being end of June, there was not much traffic. The only thing hard was, traveling east, the sun was quite strong on my side. But I put a towel on the door window and that helped a lot. I am looking forward to go for a swim later on this evening.'

'Are you plotting against us or is it just girls chatter?

'No Carl! Ida was telling me about your driving skills and impatience on the road. But I defended you as much as I could.'

The four of them sat in the shade under the vines sipping cold drinks and relaxing.

After dinner and a short rest, a fifteen minute walk took them to the beach close enough to Marcelo's boat.

'This is what I miss on our beeches', said Ida. 'Warm sea! It must be well over twenty!

'I think Marcelo mentioned it was about twenty five or so. I am not sure myself.'

After a few days doing nothing but swimming and sunbathing during the day and going out for a meal in the evening Marcelo took Carl fishing but they found it too warm and a cruise round a few islands sounded much more attractive.

For Marcelo and Carl the swimming started first thing in the morning, continued during the day and they swam just before they retired for the night. There was a grill installed at the side of the boat and it was up to the men to catch fish and to grill it. There were many places where they could purchase fresh fruit and knowing it had not been sprayed, gave extra pleasure. The cruise lasted four days but it seemed it passed in a flash.

Carl and Marcelo walked to the house to bring the car as there were many things to be brought back to the house. Just as they brought the car down to the marina, Ida shouted from the boat.

'Carl your mobile rang but by the time I found it it stopped. Here it is!

Carl looked at the number on the screen and said.

'It is our neighbour. I wonder what is he calling about.'

After talking on his mobile for a few minutes, Carl looked somewhat agitated and finally spoke.

'Ida, we have been burgled. My God it is, as far as I know, the very first break in in our neighbourhood.'

'What did Alain say Carl? Asked Ida.

'Just that! They noticed our back door open and when they went to have a look, it was definitely a break in. As far as they could see the only place in the house burgled was my office. Everything else appears in order.'

'I am sorry my friend. It must worry you being so far away.'

'We will have to cut our holidays short Tania. Said Ida. 'Carl what about leaving tomorrow morning?

'I was thinking of that as well. But let us take this stuff to the house first. Here Marcelo! You pass me the bags and I will fill the car.'

Next morning Carl and Ida said farewell to their hosts and drove off worrying of what will they find on their arrival home.

It has never happened before.

Three boys, triplets to be precise, in hospital, having same symptoms but it is not a decease and it is not contagious. How on earth did this happen?

After doing numerous tests, two young consultants suggested to send the boy's DNA to be analysed by a powerful computer in the USA. The senior consultant rejected the idea but after a few days, when the media interest suddenly appeared the consultant "suggested" and then decided to contact the appropriate people in the USA with the aim to send them the three DNA samples to be analysed, compared and to be searched for a possible reason linking the symptoms of the triplets.

It took two whole weeks for the work by the world famous computer to present a possible link.

Premature ageing, was the suggested answer.

Another two weeks and another statement from the computer:

Telomer

Telomer, is a region of highly repetitive DNA at the end of a linear chromosome .

During cell division, a small piece of the telomer is consumed. In humans, the shortening of Telomers is strongly correlated with aging. The shortening of Telomers acts, apparently as a natural defence against cancer.

The computer pointed out that a study suggested an individual's age could be estimated from the length of the Telomer.

Healthy human cell are mortal because they can divide only a finite number of times, growing older each time. Thus cells in an elderly human are much older than cells in an infant.

Telomers work as a "clock" that regulates how many times an invidual cell can divide.

'Doctor', asked the three mothers, almost in unison:

'You mentioned a clock. Could the clock be, somehow, stopped?

'Yes and no!, replied the senior consultant Mr O'Hare.

'You see, in the laboratory, cells in tissue with introduction of telemetries have extended the length of telomers and so extended the number the cells could divide. But there is a problem.

In humans, if we introduce telemetries, all germ cells and all cancer cells will be activated as well and the time when scientists will be able to selectively introduce telemetries is still very far from being realized.

Research on clinical telemetries is currently focused on the development of methods for the accurate diagnosis of cancer and on novel anti-telemetries cancer terapeutics. I am so sorry I could not give you any hope.'

'Could you give us any indication of what to expect please? Asked Amanda in a voice so weak that Mr O'Hare could just about understand what she asked.

'I am afraid I can not. You see there has never been a case like this. Because here are three almost identical cases, the only explanation I could think of is that there must have been an accident during the IVF treatment, either aided or unaided.

I am so sorry.'

'Hello! Said Carl after rushing through the front door on Sunday afternoon.

Hello Mr Campbell, this is Claire, Mathew's wife.

Oh hello Claire. I was just thinking of calling you.

How is Mathew?

Instead the answer, he heard a cry. The only thing he could do was to wait for Claire to calm down.

Mr Campbell, Mathew is not well. The three brothers went to London and they, the doctors, sent their DNA samples to the USA and the results of the analysis were very bad. I fear thet Mathew, and his two brothers as well, have not long left to live. According to the consultant there they are about three times their chronological age. I will write you a letter and enclose details of the hospital test results. I am sorry to bother you but you were so good to Mathew and me when we visited you and Mrs Campbell.'

Monday morning there was another call, this time from Mr Atkinson.

'Mr Campbell. Do you have copies of the stuff you sent me last month please?

'Actually I don't Mr Atkinson. While my wife and

myself were on holidays, our house was broken in and we were robbed but, believe it or not, the only think stolen was the copies of our correspondence and the electronic gear my friend Marcelo retrieved from the site of the old Clinic.'

'Oh my God. We had a break in with the same result and not only that. My colleague, Mr Thorp was found dead in the south of Spain. It appears that the forces of evil are still on the alert. Is there anything else we can do concerning the case?

'I am afraid there is nothing left Mr Atkinson. I am sorry.'

Next Carl decided to phone Marcelo.

'0208' uttered Marcelo lifting the receiver.

Marcelo its me, Carl.'

'Hello Carl! Ida was talking to Tania this morning say-ing something of yours was stolen only. What was that about?

'Well, there has been a clean up. Marcelo. The only thing stolen here was my correspondence with Mr Atkinson and the gear you left here. Absolutely nothing else.'

'I smell a rat there.' interrupted Marcelo.

'And a big one it seems. Mr Atkinson's Clinic has been broken in and the only thing stolen was his correspondence with me. And there is more. Mr Thorp has been found in Spain, it appears poisoned although not yet confirmed.'

'I am sorry Carl. And I am sorry for the three boys and their mothers and the young Claire, Mathew's wife. I believe this is the end of the line. But Carl listen! The weather here is still hot. Why don't you and Ida come again. There are many cheap flights and plenty of time to go fishing. What do you say?

'Maybe we will Marcelo. If you hear from me soon that'll mean we are coming.'